PHARMACOLOGY
NCLEX-RN REVIEW:

100 Practice Questions with Detailed
Rationales Explaining Correct & Incorrect
Answer Choices

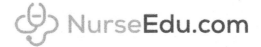

Disclaimer:

FREE BONUS

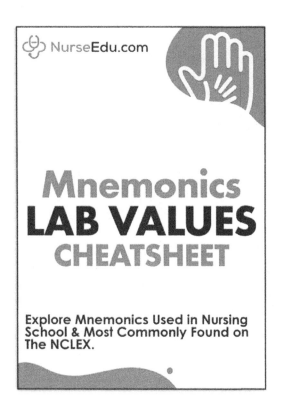

FREE Download – Just Visit:

NurseEdu.com/bonus

TABLE OF CONTENTS

CHAPTER 1:

NCLEX-RN – PHARMACOLOGY – 100 QUESTIONS

Multiple Choice

1. A 75-year-old patient is being started on digoxin and requires education on the medication. Which of the following patient statements indicates an understanding of the instructions for how to take digoxin?

    A. "I will take it at the same time every day and store it at room temperature."

    B. "1 understand that I should notify my health care provider if my heart seems to be beating too slowly or if I experience enlarged breasts."

    C. "I understand that I should call my doctor if I experience nausea, vomiting, or confusion."

D. "As soon as I realize I missed a dose, I will take it to keep my blood levels stable."

Rationale:

Correct answer: A

Digoxin is a digitalis glycoside used for the treatment of CHF, atrial fibrillation, atrial flutter, and tachycardia. It is most important that the patient and his wife understand the correct way to take digoxin in order to prevent serious side effects. Direct verbalization of understanding is the best way for the nurse to determine if the patient education has been successful. Important for the patient to know: take at the same time every day and store at room temperature. It can cause many serious side effects, including hypotension, bradycardia, dizziness, and mental disturbances.

B is incorrect because although bradycardia and enlarged breasts (in men) are adverse effects of digoxin, knowing the adverse effects does not demonstrate knowledge of how to correctly take the medication.

C is incorrect because although these are signs of digoxin toxicity, this does not demonstrate knowledge of how to correctly take the medication.

D is incorrect because the client should be taught to take a missed dose as soon as they remember <u>unless the next</u>

<u>dose is scheduled within 12 hours.</u> Do not stop the medication suddenly.

2. The nurse is instructing the client recently diagnosed with hypertension about starting oral captopril. Due to the potential side effects of early therapy with this medication, which nursing diagnosis is appropriate for this patient?

    A. Activity intolerance
    B. Risk for injury
    C. Disturbed body image
    D. Self-care deficit

Rationale:

Correct answer: B

Captopril, like all other angiotensin-converting enzyme (ACE) inhibitors, frequently causes hypotension when therapy is initiated. This is known as the first-dose effect. The patient must be taught to call for help before getting out of bed or rising from a chair to prevent orthostatic hypotension, which is a risk for falls. Another common side effect of ACE inhibitors is a dry cough. This does not occur in all patients and is not necessarily a reason to stop the medication. Note: the first-dose effect does not occur with all anti-hypertensives.

A is incorrect because although ACE inhibitors can initially cause hypotension, the patient usually is able to return to previous levels of activity once accommodated to the medication.

C is incorrect because there is no relationship between ACE inhibitors and body image.

D is incorrect because there is no relationship between ACE inhibitors and patients' ability to care for themselves.

3. The healthcare provider has ordered atenolol 25 mg once daily at 0900 for a patient. Which is the correct action the nurse should take?

   A. Administer the drug by the transdermal route.
   B. Administer the drug by mouth (PO).
   C. Administer the drug by intravenous route (IV).
   D. Contact the healthcare provider to clarify the route.

Rationale:

Correct answer: D

The medication order "Atenolol 25 mg once daily at 0900" is missing the route of administration. The healthcare provider must be notified in order to clarify the route. Never assume the route on a medication order as different routes usually require different dosages due to the mechanism of action, onset of action, and duration of action. Atenolol can be administered as a tablet orally, as a liquid suspension for administration through a feeding tube, as a patch for transdermal delivery, or as intravenous medication.

A is incorrect because the original order does not state the transdermal route.

B is incorrect because the original order does not state the oral route.

C is incorrect because the original order does not state the intravenous route.

4. The nurse is reconciling medication history for a patient. Which of the following questions will return the most pertinent information from the patient?

    A. "Do you use sleeping pills at night?"
    B. "Is there a family history of heart disease?"
    C. "When you experience pain, how do you relieve it?"
    D. "What diseases did you have as a child?"

Rationale:

Correct answer: C

Asking open-ended questions will elicit the best information from a patient when obtaining medication history as well as any other pertinent health information.

Asking the patient how he relieves pain will help the nurse provide patient-centered care and make the patient more comfortable as he is being treated.

A is incorrect because it is a closed-ended question and does not give much information regarding his medication history.

B is incorrect because it is a closed-ended question and not part of the patient's medication history.

D is incorrect because it is not pertinent to the patient's medication history.

5. A 75-year-old woman admitted with an upper respiratory tract infection informs the nurse she is allergic to penicillin. Which response by the nurse is most appropriate?

    A. "There are many people who are also allergic to penicillin."

    B. "Because this medication is given so frequently, your allergy is not a major concern."

    C. "When did you take penicillin, and what reaction did you have?"

    D. "Older patients don't usually have drug reactions because of built-up resistance."

Rationale:

Correct answer: C

Many patients confuse side effects with allergic reactions. Asking the patient what type of reaction she had (and when) will help clarify whether the reaction was truly allergic or a side effect to the penicillin. Using an open-ended question will provide the best information. True signs of allergy to penicillin include skin rash, hives, itching, wheezing, or shortness of breath. These signs often occur with hours of the first dose but can actually occur even after the entire 7-10-day course of the medication has been completed. Diarrhea, nausea, headache, and vaginal itching are side effects of penicillin but no signs of allergy.

A is incorrect because it does not elicit any further information from the patient. This response is dismissive and is not patient-focused. Be sure to select an answer that keeps the focus on the patient in the question.

B is incorrect because an allergy is always of concern when administering medications.

D is incorrect because the immune system does not build up resistance to allergic reactions.

6. A patient newly diagnosed with type 2 diabetes mellitus has been prescribed metformin by the healthcare

provider. Which of the following statements by the nurse is most appropriate regarding how to take metformin?

A. "This medication will cure your type 2 diabetes."

B. "Have some juice or candy available if you feel weak or dizzy after taking your metformin."

C. "These extended-release tablets can be crushed and mixed with juice or pudding to help you swallow it."

D. "Do not take the metformin with food as it will decrease absorption and effectiveness of the medication."

Rationale:

Correct answer: B

Metformin works by decreasing the production of glucose by the liver as well as decreasing absorption of glucose and improving sensitivity to insulin. This could potentially lead to hypoglycemia. The best course of action is to instruct the patient to have some source of glucose like juice or candy to prevent weakness and dizziness felt when hypoglycemia occurs.

A is incorrect because metformin does not cure type 2 diabetes but improves glucose use in the body.

C is incorrect because extended-release tablets should never be cut or crushed, as this negates the extended-release. (If the client is unable to swallow the metformin tablet whole, a specific form of the medication can be prescribed, which comes in powdered packets for mixing with food.)

D is incorrect because ingestion of food with metformin does not affect how the drug is absorbed or how it works. It is best to have a meal soon after taking metformin in order to prevent hypoglycemia.

7. The nurse discusses medication history with the patient. The patient tells the nurse, "I take aspirin occasionally for headaches but didn't mention that before, since it is non-prescription." What is the best response by the nurse?

   A. "True, over-the-counter medications, in general, are not harmful."
   B. "Aspirin is a safe drug. I'm more concerned about prescription medications."
   C. "Even though aspirin is over-the-counter, we still need to know how much you take and how often"
   D. "You need to be honest about all medications and drugs you take. Are there other medications you have not informed us of?"

Rationale:

Correct answer: C

It is important to obtain information on all medications, both prescription and non-prescription, as well as over-the-counter and herbal supplements. Knowing everything the patient takes can help identify any medication interactions. Aspirin can contribute to bleeding tendencies and works synergistically with medications such as anti-thrombotics. Aspirin is also contraindicated for patients with thrombocytopenia, hepatic dysfunction, renal disease, and pregnancy.

A is incorrect because it is a false generalized statement.

B is incorrect because of the potential for bleeding and liver damage.

D is incorrect because it could prevent open communication and inhibits patient-centered care. Starting statements with the word "you" is non-therapeutic. Use caution when asking questions; be sure to be non-confrontational.

8. A patient is visited by the home health nurse after recently being discharged from the hospital. The patient is wearing a small mesh pouch with a strong odor on her chest and has herbal tea at her side. The patient tells the nurse that her grandmother suggested herbal treatments to help her "get better." What is the best response by the nurse?

A. "If you want to feel better, you should do what the doctor said."
B. "What are the ingredients in the tea and the pack? Do you use them often?"
C. "Herbal remedies often are contraindicated with prescription medications."
D. "Have you been taking your medications as prescribed?"

Rationale:

Correct answer: B

The nurse needs more information at this time. Not all herbal remedies are dangerous. Herbal supplements and home remedies can be useful for some patients, but it is important to know what is in them to identify potential interactions with prescription medications.

A is incorrect because it does not encourage open communication with the patient. It is non-therapeutic to tell a patient, "you *should...*"

C is incorrect because it does not encourage communication with the patient and patient-centered care. Although this is a true statement, it does not address the therapeutic nurse-patient relationship. It is better at this time to assess what remedies the client is using and determine if there are any contraindications with prescribed medications.

D is incorrect because it prevents open communication with the patient regarding home remedies. Although this is an important question to ask, it's a greater priority to ask about the herbal ingredients, which is the topic of the question.

9. A patient is in the clinic for a check-up and tells the nurse he has used herbal supplements containing kava for 3 years for relaxation at night. He appears to be slightly jaundiced. The nurse advises him to stop taking the herbal supplements and see the healthcare provider. What else should be done by the nurse?

    A. Report the incident to MedWatch.
    B. Notify the State Pharmaceutical Board.
    C. Contact the Nursing Supervisor.
    D. No further action is required.

Rationale:

Correct answer: A

Jaundice is the buildup of bilirubin, a product of red blood cell destruction, in the skin and sclera as a result of excess red blood cell destruction, liver failure, or obstruction of biliary passage. The cause of this patient's jaundice needs to be identified. MedWatch was established by the FDA to track drug therapy adverse events and problems.

B is incorrect because the State Pharmaceutical Board does not monitor herbal supplements.

C is incorrect because this situation is not an indication to use the vertical chain of command. The nurse should use the chain of command when administrative or safety issues have been identified.

D is incorrect because the cause of the patient's jaundice needs to be identified before any further health issues arise.

10. The nurse is caring for a patient experiencing severe pain due to pathologic spinal fractures from metastatic bone cancer. The dosing schedule for administration of this patient's pain medication would best be scheduled for:

    A. PRN
    B. Around the clock
    C. When the patient is awake only
    D. Around the clock and PRN

    Rationale:

    Correct answer: D

Patients with cancer are usually prescribed long-acting opioids and experience opioid tolerance, causing analgesic effects to wear off. This causes breakthrough pain between scheduled doses, requiring additional PRN doses to effectively manage pain.

A is incorrect because a sufficient level of pain medication cannot be maintained with PRN dosing, leading to ineffective pain management. Bone cancer is considered to be extremely painful. The nurse should not wait until the patient complains of pain to offer medication.

B is incorrect because, over time, the patient may become tolerant of opioids, causing analgesic effects to wear off and leading to breakthrough pain. PRN meds are needed as well (such as PO fast-acting liquid morphine).

C is incorrect because the patient may awaken with pain, leading to ineffective pain management and disrupted sleep-wake cycles.

11. The nurse cares for a post-operative patient with an opioid PCA pump for pain management. The nurse finds the patient unresponsive to voice, respirations 8 BPM, and blood pressure 98/54 mmHg. Once the PCA is stopped, what is the next action the nurse should perform?

    A. Notify the charge nurse

B. Draw arterial blood gases

C. Administer an opiate antagonist

D. Perform a thorough physical assessment and neurological check

Rationale:

Correct answer: C

Opioid antagonists such as Naloxone reverse the effects of opioid analgesia as well as CNS and respiratory depression. These are standard orders when opioids are administered, especially when a PCA is in use.

A is incorrect because immediate patient care at the bedside is the priority. It is important to notify the charge nurse after providing immediate care to reverse the effect of the opioid.

B is incorrect because although an ABG may confirm hypoxia, it is not a priority for the nurse to assess this patient any further at this time. The nurse has enough data; intervention is necessary. (Also, ABG results will take time to return. The nurse should do something *now*.)

D is incorrect because the assessment is not the priority right now. After administering the antagonist, the nurse should monitor the patient's respiratory rate and BP, looking for an increase in both. Then a thorough physical assessment and neurological check can be performed.

12. A patient has been prescribed transdermal fentanyl patches for bone pain related to metastatic cancer. When the patient asks about the benefits of these patches, the best response should include which of the following?

    A. "Transdermal fentanyl patches deliver more constant levels of the drug for pain relief."

    B. "You will experience less constipation and dry mouth with transdermal fentanyl patches."

    C. "Drowsiness is less of a problem with transdermal fentanyl patches than with oral opioids."

    D. "This medication patch has a lower potential for dependency than with other pain medications."

Rationale:

Correct answer: A

Transdermal fentanyl patches can provide pain relief for up to 7 days. The medication is delivered constantly, maintaining effective levels in the bloodstream for pain control. However, these are not effective for the dose titration, so they are used after stable analgesia is achieved.

B is incorrect because this form of opioid administered can still lead to constipation and dry mouth.

C is incorrect because this form of opioid administered can still lead to drowsiness.

D is incorrect because this form of opioid administered can still lead to dependency and other adverse effects.

13. The nurse on the medical unit is caring for four patients who have acetaminophen ordered for pain. When reviewing charts, the nurse determines which patient should not receive acetaminophen?

    A. Patient with fever 102.9°F (39.2°C)
    B. Patient admitted for DVT
    C. Patient admitted for severe hepatitis
    D. Patient recovering from abdominal surgery 3 days ago

Rationale:

Correct answer: C

Acetaminophen is metabolized by the liver. Severe hepatitis and liver disease are contraindications to the administration of this medication because it can lead to toxicity.

A is incorrect because a fever is an indication of an antipyretic such as acetaminophen.

B is incorrect because DVT is not a contraindication for acetaminophen. Acetaminophen may actually be the best pain medication for a DVT patient, especially if they are receiving a blood-thinner, such as heparin. (Ibuprofen for pain would increase the risk for bleeding on a client who is receiving a clot-buster or blood-thinner.)

D is incorrect because post-abdominal surgery is not a contraindication for acetaminophen.

14. The nurse is caring for four patients on the surgical unit. The medical records are reviewed for all four patients. Which of the following patients should not receive an opioid analgesic medication?

    A. Patient with renal insufficiency related to renal calculi
    B. Patient with severe asthma
    C. Patient in balanced skeletal traction awaiting surgery for splinting of left femur
    D. Patient with diabetes mellitus

Rationale:

Correct answer: B

Opioids are known CNS depressants that can cause respiratory depression. This is more common in patients who have a history of respiratory compromise, including asthma. Additionally, patients with chronic obstructive pulmonary disease and sleep apnea should be administered an alternate medication. Other instances in which the nurse should question opioid therapy include a history of substance abuse, pregnancy, suspected illegal activity, and brain trauma.

A is incorrect because renal insufficiency is not a contraindication for opioid analgesics. Morphine and hydromorphone are commonly used to treat the pain associated with kidney stones.

C is incorrect because skeletal traction is not a contraindication for opioid medications. Skeletal traction is often very painful. Administration of analgesics and antispasmodics are part of the treatment plan.

D is incorrect because diabetes mellitus is not a contraindication for opioid analgesics.

15. The surgical charge nurse is reviewing the cases scheduled for surgery. Which of the following patients is at increased risk for complications from general anesthesia?

    A. 74-year-old female scheduled for hip replacement
    B. 48-year-old male who is physically active and quit smoking ten years ago
    C. 6-year-old female in good health with no prior anesthesia
    D. 40-year-old female scheduled for laser vision correction

Rationale:

Correct answer: A

Older patients are at higher risk for complications following general anesthesia due to decreased ability of the liver to metabolize anesthesia and risk for impaired renal function in clearing metabolites from the bloodstream. This can lead to longer recovery time, respiratory system depression, and gastrointestinal system side effects.

B is incorrect because the patient is no longer smoking and physically active. The residual effects from smoking are not as great a risk factor as the age in patient A.

C is incorrect because the patient is healthy, although close monitoring would be necessary as a reaction to anesthesia is unknown.

D is incorrect because the patient has an outpatient procedure, and lower doses of anesthesia will be administered.

16. A patient is in the post-anesthesia care unit recovering from abdominal surgery and general anesthesia. Which of the following assessments is the nurse's greatest priority during the immediate postoperative period?

   A. Airway
   B. Pupil response to light
   C. Sensation return in the lower extremities

D. Level of consciousness

Rationale:

Correct answer: A

The airway is of the highest importance during the immediate recovery phase from general anesthesia. General anesthesia suppresses the respiratory center of the CNS, which interferes with the ability to maintain a patent airway and respirations within normal limits. The nurse should assess airway patency and spontaneous breathing. Oxygen saturation levels should be evaluated by continuous pulse-ox monitoring in the immediate post-op period.

B is incorrect because pupillary reflexes are an indication of the level of consciousness, but the airway is a greater priority.

C is incorrect because it is of concern to monitor but not the main concern. Residual paresthesia or paralysis are not common complications with general anesthesia, and the airway is more important.

D is incorrect because assessing the airway is a greater priority. To assess LOC, the nurse evaluates orientation and level of responsiveness using the Glascow Coma Scale: eye-opening response, verbal response, and motor response.

17. A 22-year-old man is admitted to the emergency department for oral benzodiazepine overdose. He is responsive but drowsy. Which immediate intervention will the nurse implement?

    A. Hemodialysis for removal of the benzodiazepine

    B. Administration of flumazenil 0.2 mg IV over 30 seconds

    C. Administration of naloxone 10 mg IV

    D. Intubation and mechanical ventilation

Rationale:

Correct answer: A

Flumazenil is a benzodiazepine antidote that reverses sedative effects and binds at receptors in the CNS. It is used for oral overdose as well as intravenous sedation. It is important for the nurse to initiate seizure precautions after administering this antidote because patients who are withdrawing from benzodiazepines are at risk for seizures.

B is incorrect because the priority is to administer the flumazenil IV. Hemodialysis will not reverse the benzodiazepine action. However, once the patient is stabilized, hemodialysis may be indicated to clear the benzodiazepine from the patient's circulation.

C is incorrect because naloxone is administered for opioid overdose, not benzodiazepine overdose. Furthermore, the dose of naloxone is generally 0.4-2 mg IV every two minutes until a max of 10 mg or reversal of symptoms is reached.

D is incorrect because the patient is responsive and able to maintain his own airway. Intubation may become necessary if the flumazenil does not increase the patient's level of consciousness. The nurse should have the crash cart nearby and be prepared to call the health care provider in the event that intubation is needed. It is not within the nurse's scope of practice to intubate a patient.

18. The nurse is teaching a patient about the use of zaleplon. Which of the following patient statements indicates an understanding?

    A. "I should take this medication 1 hour before bedtime with a snack."
    B. "I should take this medication immediately before bedtime."
    C. "I may experience morning drowsiness with this medication."
    D. "I understand that I should limit my alcohol consumption to no more than 2 drinks daily while on this medication."

Rationale:

Correct answer: B

Zaleplon is a short-acting miscellaneous hypnotic drug that shares characteristics with benzodiazepines. Patients are advised to take this medication immediately before going to bed.

A is incorrect because zaleplon has a rapid onset and helps mostly with difficulty falling asleep. Due to its extremely short half-life, it may not help reduce premature awakenings.

C is incorrect because the patient does need to be educated regarding morning drowsiness, but it is less likely to occur with this type of medication. Zolpidem is more likely to cause morning drowsiness.

D is incorrect because combining the medication with alcohol will have a synergistic effect. Alcohol should completely be avoided while taking this medication.

19. A patient in the medical unit tells the nurse she is having trouble sleeping. Which is the first action the nurse should take to address the problem?

    A. Administer a sedative-hypnotic medication
    B. Offer herbal valerian tea
    C. Encourage exercise during the hospital stay
    D. Provide a restful, quiet environment

Rationale:

Correct answer: D

A quiet environment that is conducive to sleep is the first intervention a nurse should attempt when a patient is having trouble sleeping. The nurse may need to close the curtains, turn off the lights and television, restrict visitors, silence equipment, and cluster care in order to help the patient rest.

A is incorrect because a nonpharmacological method should be attempted first.

B is incorrect because herbal supplements often interact with other medications.

C is incorrect because providing a quiet environment for rest is more important than activity. Once the patient's sleep-wake cycle has been addressed, the nurse can encourage activity as tolerated.

20. A patient is being discharged after a total hysterectomy and is prescribed zolpidem 10 mg at bedtime PRN. What is the priority action the nurse should take?

    A. Review possible adverse effects with the patient
    B. Suggest a glass of wine at bedtime
    C. Contact the healthcare provider to verify the dosage
    D. Assist with locating a pharmacy for filling the prescription

Rationale:

Correct answer: C

Zolpidem is a short-acting nonbenzodiazepine hypnotic that is often prescribed as a sleep aide. The FDA recommends a maximum dose of 5 mg of zolpidem QHS for women due to potential impairment the following morning. The nurse should contact the healthcare provider to verify the dosage before discharging the patient.

A is incorrect because although it is important to review adverse effects, it is not the priority action. The safest option is to question the dosage ordered.

B is incorrect because alcohol has additive effects with CNS depressants such as zolpidem. The nurse should educate the patient that alcohol should be avoided while taking this medication.

D is incorrect because it is not the priority action. This is more of a psychosocial answer choice. Clarifying the dose ordered is a more physical priority and helps the nurse provide safe patient care.

21. The healthcare provider has ordered modafinil to treat a patient with narcolepsy. Which adverse effect would the nurse monitor for?

A. Bradycardia and dilute urine

B. Nervousness and black, tarry stools

C. Mental clouding

D. Nighttime drowsiness and palpitations

Rationale:

Correct Answer: B

Narcolepsy is a neurologic condition that causes patients to fall asleep unexpectedly during normal daily activities. It is an incurable condition that can be treated with CNS stimulants (such as modafinil, methylphenidate and amphetamine), which work similarly to the sympathetic nervous system, affecting the CNS and respiratory systems primarily. Common effects of CNS stimulants include mood elevation, increased alertness, and decreased fatigue. Due to the similarity of sympathetic nervous system stimulation, patients can adversely exhibit nervousness. Black, tarry stools are another side effect of this medication.

A is incorrect because sympathetic nervous stimulation causes tachycardia and has no known effect on the concentration of urine.

C is incorrect because modafinil increases alertness.

D is incorrect because although modafinil can cause palpitations, it is more likely to cause insomnia than drowsiness.

22. A patient is beginning treatment with sumatriptan. When providing patient teaching regarding the administration of the medication, which information should the nurse include?

    A. Correct intravenous injection technique
    B. Take medication before worsening of headache
    C. Allow 30 minutes between injections
    D. Do not exceed 400 mg PO per 24-hour period

Rationale:

Correct answer: B

Sumatriptan is a serotonin receptor agonist causing vasoconstriction and relief of headache symptoms when taken after a headache has started. PO form is available in 25, 50, and 100 mg tablets, and the max dosage is 200 mg per day.

A is incorrect because sumatriptan is available as a nasal spray, PO medication, and subcutaneous injection. This medication should not be given intravenously because of the potential for coronary vasospasm.

C is incorrect because when given subcutaneously, the maximum dose in 24 hours is 6mg given a minimum of one hour apart.

D is incorrect because the max dosage is 40 mg of nasal spray per 24 hours or 200 mg of PO medication per 24 hours.

23. A patient is ordered intravenous phenytoin for seizure prevention. The nurse knows which of the following is the most appropriate action?

    A. IV doses are given by rapid push

    B. Administer in normal saline solution

    C. Administer in a dextrose solution

    D. Continuous infusion of the medication

Rationale:

Correct answer: B

Phenytoin can only be diluted in normal saline. A filter is used for IV infusion to prevent any precipitates from infusing into the patient's circulation.

A is incorrect because phenytoin must be administered by slow IV push to prevent inflammation and adverse effects, including cardiac arrest.

C is incorrect because phenytoin can only be diluted in normal saline.

D is incorrect because phenytoin is irritating to veins and can only be given by slow IV push or PO. When giving this medication PO, the nurse should keep in mind that phenytoin is highly protein-bound, so it should not be taken with food. Tube feeding should be held for 20 to 30 minutes before and after the nurse administers phenytoin suspension.

24. The nurse is preparing to administer carbamazepine to four clients. Which of the following would concern the nurse the most?

    A. The patient has a history of heart failure and is scheduled to receive his digoxin loading dose today
    B. The patient who is requesting acetaminophen for a headache
    C. The patient who is on day four of a 7-day treatment of ampicillin for a bacterial infection
    D. The patient who takes warfarin and has a hemoglobin of 13g/dL

Rationale:

Correct answer: B

Carbamazepine is an anticonvulsant that works by decreasing the nerve impulses that cause seizures.

Concomitant usage of carbamazepine and acetaminophen can increase the risk of toxicity with acetaminophen and reduce the efficacy of carbamazepine.

A is incorrect because there is no interaction with digoxin. History of heart failure is not a contraindication to carbamazepine use.

C is incorrect because there is no contraindication or interaction between penicillin drugs and carbamazepine.

D is incorrect because there is no interaction with warfarin. Carbamazepine can cause decreased bone marrow activity, so hemoglobin levels should be monitored. This patient has normal hemoglobin, so this is not a concern.

25. A patient taking phenytoin has lab drawn, and his level is found to be 26 mcg/mL. What symptom would the nurse expect to see in a patient with this phenytoin level?

   A. Poor control of muscle movements
   B. BP 180/98 and HR 54 bpm
   C. Seizures
   D. No symptoms; this is a therapeutic level

Rationale:

Correct answer: A

Phenytoin is administered to manage tonic-clonic and partial seizures as a first-line drug. Therapeutic levels of this medication range between 10 and 20 mcg/mL. Increased levels cause nystagmus (rapid, involuntary eye movements), ataxia (poor muscular control), dysarthria (motor speech disorder), and encephalopathy.

B is incorrect because increased levels of phenytoin do not cause hypertension and bradycardia.

C is incorrect because seizures are a symptom of decreased levels of phenytoin in the blood, not increased.

D is incorrect because the therapeutic range is 10-20 mcg/mL.

26. A patient is admitted to the medical unit with a history of seizures. During the physical assessment, the nurse notes a generalized seizure that lasts several minutes. Which drug does the nurse anticipate administering?

   A. Valproic acid
   B. Gabapentin
   C. Carbamazepine
   D. Diazepam

Rationale:

Correct answer: D

Diazepam is administered for anxiety, alcohol withdrawal, seizures, and as a skeletal muscle relaxant. It can also be given as preoperative medication. It is one drug of choice for status epilepticus, a condition in which multiple seizures occur without breaks between, which can cause hypotension, hypoxia, brain damage, and even death.

A is incorrect because valproic acid is for the long-term management of seizures, not status epilepticus. This is the agent of choice for many seizure disorders in young children. When administering valproic acid, the nurse should monitor bleeding time, liver studies, and platelets.

B is incorrect because gabapentin is for long-term management of seizures, not status epilepticus. When administering gabapentin, the nurse should monitor weight and mood changes.

C is incorrect because carbamazepine is for the long-term management of partial seizures and tonic-clonic seizures. (Remember that carbamazepine interacts with grapefruit juice.)

27. A patient has been prescribed an antiepileptic medication for the first time. After the nurse educates the patient regarding the medication, which patient statement indicates the need for further education?

   A. "The medication needs to be taken at the same time daily."

B. "If I need to take over-the-counter medications, I will check with the healthcare provider first."

C. "I will keep bloodwork appointments as scheduled."

D. "Once my drug levels are therapeutic, I will be able to drive myself."

Rationale:

Correct answer: D

Many antiepileptic medications have CNS effects, including drowsiness and visual disturbances, especially when a medication is initiated. Driving regulations vary from state to state, so the Department of Motor Vehicles should be contacted regarding regulations. Most states require at least a 1-year period seizure-free before driving alone.

A is incorrect because seizure medication should be taken at the same time daily to maintain blood levels. This is a true statement indicating an understanding of the instructions.

B is incorrect because over-the-counter medications can interact with antiepileptics, so checking with the healthcare provider is correct, indicating an understanding of the instructions.

C is incorrect because blood work should be monitored regularly to maintain therapeutic blood levels of the medication, indicating an understanding of the instructions.

28. A patient with Parkinson's disease is taking entacapone. Which intervention by the nurse is appropriate for this patient?

    A. Educate the patient that discoloration of the urine is common with this medication.
    B. Tell the patient to limit intake of tyramine-containing foods.
    C. Monitor renal panel studies due to renal effects of the medication.
    D. Encourage the patient to drink fluids for dehydration prevention.

Rationale:

Correct answer: A

Parkinson's is believed to be an imbalance of dopamine and acetylcholine, and drug therapy increases dopamine and antagonizes acetylcholine to slow the progression of the disease. Entacapone is a COMT inhibitor whose side effects include discoloration of the urine. Entacapone is often used as a combination drug to enhance levodopa and carbidopa.

B is incorrect because limiting the intake of tyramine applies to MAO-I medications because of the risk for hypertensive crisis. (Foods that contain tyramine include: aged cheese, beer, pickled products, salami, bouillon, and soy sauce.)

C is incorrect because entacapone does not have serious renal effects. Common side effects include abdominal pain, nausea, vomiting, fatigue, and dry mouth.

D is incorrect because dehydration is not a side effect of entacapone. While encouraging fluids is generally good patient education, this does not apply directly to entacapone.

29. A patient is educated by the nurse regarding antiparkinson medications. Which of the following statements should be included by the nurse?

    A. "When your tremors and weakness improve, the dosage will be reduced."
    B. "If you miss a dose, take double at the next dose to maintain blood levels of the medication."
    C. "Notify your healthcare provider immediately if you note a brown or orange color to your urine."
    D. "Change positions slowly, so your blood pressure does not drop."

Rationale:

Correct answer: D

Many antiparkinson medications cause hypotension and orthostatic hypotension due to dopaminergic stimulation, so the patient should be educated to change positions slowly to prevent a sudden drop in blood pressure.

A is incorrect because blood levels of the medication must be maintained in order to slow the progression of Parkinson's.

B is incorrect because increased blood levels of antiparkinson medications can cause toxicity and serious adverse effects.

C is incorrect because not all antiparkinson medications cause discoloration of the urine. This only applies if educating about entacapone. (The health care provider does not need to be notified immediately because it is an expected side effect of entacapone.)

30. A patient is admitted to the emergency room for opioid withdrawal. Which medication does the nurse anticipate administering?

    A. Amphetamine
    B. Clonidine
    C. Diazepam
    D. Disulfiram

Rationale:

Correct answer: B

Clonidine is an antihypertensive medication that can also be given to treat opioid withdrawal for up to a week. The patient's blood pressure should be checked before administration of each dose, and the clonidine should be withheld if the patient is hypotensive. The nurse must caution the patient that clonidine can cause sleepiness, dry mouth, and upset stomach.

A is incorrect because amphetamine will worsen withdrawal symptoms.

C is incorrect because diazepam will mask symptoms and potentially cause respiratory depression. Diazepam is a benzodiazepine that is sometimes used to treat alcohol withdrawal, seizures, and anxiety.

D is incorrect because disulfiram is administered for alcoholics who wish to curb the desire to drink. This medication causes unpleasant side effects when combined with alcohol.

31. A patient admitted for possible substance abuse is assessed by the nurse. Which of the following findings would indicate the use of amphetamines?

    A. Fatigue and lethargy
    B. Cardiovascular depression

C. Euphoria

D. Constipation and dysphagia

Rationale:

Correct answer: C

Amphetamines are stimulant drugs that lead to wakefulness, mood elevation and euphoria, talkativeness, alertness, and increased motor and speech activity.

A is incorrect because amphetamines are stimulants. Fatigue and lethargy may be signs of alcohol or opiate use.

B is incorrect because amphetamines are stimulants, leading to hypertension and tachycardia, not cardiovascular depression.

D is incorrect because amphetamines may increase GI motility when the smooth muscles of the intestines are relaxed.

32. A patient is receiving treatment with a beta-1 agonist medication. Which finding indicates to the nurse that the treatment is effective?

    A. Stronger heartbeat with an improved ejection fraction

    B. Heart rate decreases from 72 bpm to 59 bpm

    C. Decreased crackles are heard in the lungs

D. Increased GI motility

Rationale:

Correct answer: A

Beta-1 receptors are located in the heart. When a beta-1 agonist is used, expect to find increased heart rate, blood pressure, and contractility. Examples include: dobutamine and epinephrine.

B is incorrect because beta-1 agonists will increase heart rate and do not cause bradycardia.

C is incorrect because beta-1 agonists do not specifically affect the pulmonary system. While decreased crackles are a good outcome for the client, this is not an outcome of a beta-agonist. This would be an expected outcome of coughing and deep breathing or diuretic administration.

D is incorrect because beta-1 agonists do not specifically affect the GI system.

33. A patient is being treated with dobutamine for hypotension and tells the nurse he feels like his heart is skipping beats. What is the best intervention by the nurse?

    A. Continue to monitor the patient for therapeutic responses to the medication
    B. Increase the infusion rate to decrease palpitations

C. Discontinue the medication immediately

D. Assess vital signs and heart rhythm

Rationale:

Correct answer: D

Dobutamine is a beta-1 selective agonist similar to intrinsic dopamine. Stimulation of the beta-1 receptors causes increased heart rate, blood pressure, and contractility. This stimulation can cause cardiac rhythm disturbances, including palpitations, as reported by the patient. The vital signs and heart rhythm should be assessed to see if the medication rate needs to be decreased.

A is incorrect because palpitations are a side effect, not a therapeutic response to the medication. Other adverse effects are increased heart rate, hypertension, and phlebitis.

B is incorrect because increasing the infusion would cause increased palpitations.

C is incorrect because immediate discontinuation of the medication may cause reflex hypotension. Dobutamine should be tapered down slowly with careful hemodynamic monitoring.

34. The nurse is preparing to inject phentolamine subcutaneously into an area of extravasated dopamine where a patient had a peripheral IV. Which effects will the nurse expect to see?

    A. Vasoconstriction
    B. Vasodilation
    C. Analgesia
    D. Hypotension

Rationale:

Correct answer: B

Dopamine is a potent vasoconstrictor, so when phentolamine is injected (SQ) into the site, the nurse should see vasodilation in order to reverse the effects of dopamine and prevent loss of the affected extremity.

A is incorrect because phentolamine causes vasodilation.

C is incorrect because phentolamine is not an analgesic.

D is incorrect because this is a local SQ injection that does not cause hypotension. Phentolamine can be administered IV to control the hypertensive crisis, and by that route, it can cause a hypotensive reaction. Phentolamine can also be used in instances of cocaine-induced cardiovascular complications.

35. A patient is being discharged from the hospital after having experienced a myocardial infarction (MI). He has been started on therapy with nadolol. Which of the following statements should the nurse include when teaching the patient about the primary purpose of nadolol?

   A. "This medication will cause your coronary arteries to dilate."
   B. "This medication will prevent your blood pressure from getting too low."
   C. "This medication will increase the heart's conduction through the SA node."
   D. "This medication will protect your heart from catecholamines circulating in the bloodstream."

Rationale:

Correct answer: D

Beta-blockers, such as nadolol, are commonly given after myocardial infarction to decrease blood pressure, decrease heart rate, and protect the heart from catecholamines circulating in the bloodstream. Catecholamines include epinephrine, which increases heart rate and blood pressure. All of these actions decrease the workload of the heart, which is essential following myocardial infarction to prevent further infarction as well as prevent a future MI.

A is incorrect because beta-blockers do not cause coronary artery vasodilation. This would be the expected effect of nitroglycerin.

B is incorrect because it is not the main purpose of administration of a beta-blocker following MI. Beta-blockers will likely reduce the heart rate and blood pressure.

C is incorrect because a beta-blocker will slow conduction through the SA node of the heart.

36. The nurse is preparing to administer bethanechol to a postoperative patient experiencing difficulties with elimination. When educating the patient and family regarding the action of the medication, which statement does the nurse include?

   A. "The medication will decrease the tone and motility of the intestines."
   B. "The medication will increase the tone and motility of the bladder."
   C. "The full bladder sensation will be increased by this medication."

D. "The bladder sphincters will tighten, and I will be less likely to leak urine in response to this medication."

Rationale:

Correct answer: B

Bethanechol is a cholinergic agonist, or parasympathomimetic, which activates cholinergic receptors to increase motility, relax sphincters, and increase the tone of the bladder and the movement of urine. This medication can also improve gastric muscle tone and increase gastric motility.

A is incorrect because the tone and motility of the bladder and GI system will be increased by the medication.

C is incorrect because it will increase the movement of urine through the bladder, not create a full sensation. The patient likely already has a full bladder sensation, which will be alleviated with the use of bethanechol.

D is incorrect because bethanechol relaxes the sphincters of the bladder, making micturition easier. It does not help alleviate leaking urine.

37. The nurse receives an order for edrophonium. The nurse anticipates this drug is ordered for which of the following indications?

A. Alzheimer's disease symptom reduction and onset delay
B. Myasthenia gravis symptom treatment
C. Myasthenia gravis diagnosis
D. Reversal of non-depolarizing neuromuscular blocking agents post-operatively

Rationale:

Correct answer: C

Edrophonium is an indirect-acting medication that increases the concentration of acetylcholine at receptor sites, stimulating effector cells and causing contraction of skeletal muscle contraction to aid in diagnosing and treating myasthenia gravis.

A is incorrect because edrophonium is used to treat Alzheimer's disease and improve quality of life, not delay the onset or decrease symptoms. Response to this medication for this purpose has been very variable.

B is incorrect because edrophonium is used to treat myasthenia gravis, not the symptoms themselves. Symptoms of MG (muscle weakness that descends down the body beginning with the facial muscles) are commonly treated with prednisone and pyridostigmine.

D is incorrect because reversal of neuromuscular blockade is achieved with neostigmine, pyridostigmine, and physostigmine.

38. A 48-year-old man has been taking antihypertensive medication for 3 months and is in the healthcare provider's office for follow-up. He tells the nurse he has experienced difficulty with sexual intercourse. Which of the following responses by the nurse is most appropriate?

    A. "Don't worry. You'll develop a tolerance to the medication, and your symptoms will improve over time."
    B. "The healthcare provider can change either the dose or the drug."
    C. "A common side effect of this medication is sexual dysfunction. You'll learn to accept it."
    D. "Even though this is unusual, you need to stay on your medication."

Rationale:

Correct answer: B

Sexual dysfunction is a common adverse effect of antihypertensive medications and causes many patients to discontinue the medication on their own. Abrupt cessation of antihypertensives will cause rebound hypertension. These medications can be changed or the dosage decreased as long as the patient is monitored.

A is incorrect because it minimizes the patient's concern and prevents patient-centered care. This statement does not address the patient's chief complaint. It is important for the nurse to respond therapeutically to the patient's concerns and reflect a caring attitude.

C is incorrect because it prevents open communication and prevents patient-centered care. This is also a non-therapeutic response by the nurse.

D is incorrect because it is not an unusual occurrence. Many different classes of anti-hypertensive medications are available, so the healthcare provider should be notified. This patient would benefit from a change in dosage or different medication to control blood pressure.

39. A patient has been prescribed lisinopril for hypertension. When teaching the patient regarding adverse effects, which of the following statements should the nurse include?

   A. "You may experience some diarrhea while taking this medication, so be sure to drink extra fluids during the day to prevent dehydration."

   B. "If you feel like your heart is beating more slowly, please contact the healthcare provider."

C. A dry, nonproductive cough is a side effect of this medication. You can use gum or hard candy to help if this irritates you."

D. "You can expect to feel more sleepy than usual when taking this medication."

Rationale:

Correct answer: C

Angiotensin-converting enzyme inhibitors prevent angiotensin from being converted into angiotensin II, a potent vasoconstrictor. This process prevents the breakdown of bradykinin, a vasodilator, increasing the circulating concentration of bradykinin and causing the "bradykinin cough," which is a dry, nonproductive cough and an unsettling effect for some. Some patients are placed on angiotensin II receptor blockers (ARBs) to prevent this effect. Textbooks also teach that using a lozenge or chewing gum can help patients deal with this annoying symptom.

A is incorrect because ACE inhibitors do not cause diarrhea. Encouraging extra fluids for a client who is being treated for hypertension may be contraindicated.

B is incorrect because ACE inhibitors can cause tachycardia. Bradycardia is not a common side effect.

D is incorrect because ACE inhibitors do not cause drowsiness or sedation.

40. A patient has a new prescription for enalapril. Which of the following assessments would cause the nurse to monitor the patient more closely due to potential adverse effects?

  A. The patient has a history of asthma and uses a terbutaline sulfate nebulizer three times daily
  B. The patient has a history of rheumatoid arthritis and takes acetaminophen for the discomfort
  C. Hyperthyroidism
  D. Renal insufficiency

Rationale:

Correct answer: D

ACE inhibitors, such as enalapril, can lead to hyperkalemia and renal impairment. Severe heart failure patients may experience renal failure due to dependence on the renin-angiotensin-aldosterone system. Potassium levels and kidney function must be monitored closely in patients with renal insufficiency and heart failure.

A is incorrect because ACE inhibitors are not contraindicated in patients with asthma. Terbutaline sulfate does not interact with enalapril. Beta-blockers should be used cautiously with asthma patients because of the potential for bronchoconstriction.

B is incorrect because ACE inhibitors are not contraindicated for use in patients with rheumatoid arthritis. There is no interaction between ACE inhibitors and acetaminophen. ACE inhibitors can interact with NSAIDs.

C is incorrect because ACE inhibitors do not have an effect on hyperthyroidism. Medications used to treat hyperthyroidism include radioactive iodine and propylthiouracil. Neither of these interacts with ACE inhibitors.

41. The nurse is educating a patient about the appropriate use of transdermal nitroglycerin patches. Which instructions will the nurse include?

   A. "Apply the patch when you feel chest pain upon exertion."
   B. "Apply the patch at the same time every day to prevent heart palpitations."
   C. "This patch will prevent angina best if you apply it to a similar spot on your upper arm each day."
   D. "Put on a new patch daily even if you are not experiencing symptoms."

Rationale:

Correct answer: D

Nitrates are given to cause vasodilation from the relaxation of smooth muscle cells and increase blood and oxygen supply, thereby decreasing angina. Transdermal nitroglycerin patches are used to deliver a constant dose of nitrates for the above effects. A new patch should be applied daily, at the same time each day. The site should be rotated on the upper body or arms to prevent skin breakdown. Old patches should be folded in half carefully and discarded in a plastic bag where pets and other people cannot reach them, as they still may contain some active medication after disposal.

A is incorrect because nitroglycerin patches are not placed *after* exertion. The purpose of the patch is to deliver a steady dose of medication into the bloodstream for the purpose of preventing chest pain.

B is incorrect because nitroglycerin patches have no effect on the conduction system of the heart. They are not used to prevent palpitations. They should be applied at the same time every day and removed at night.

C is incorrect because although nitroglycerin patches are used to prevent angina, the site should be rotated daily to prevent skin breakdown. The patient should be instructed to select a new location each time a new patch is placed. The area should be clean and dry, with intact skin, free from irritation or thick hair.

42. The nurse is preparing intravenous nitroglycerin to be administered to a patient admitted for angina. From the nurse's knowledge, which of the following is correct regarding nitroglycerin administration?

    A. Intravenous nitroglycerin is administered IV push
    B. Dosing must be adjusted every 2 hours due to the short half-life
    C. Special tubing must be used to protect the intravenous nitroglycerin from light exposure
    D. Intravenous nitroglycerin may be administered by gravity drip infusion

Rationale:

Correct answer: C

Intravenous nitroglycerin is only given in emergency situations and through infusion pumps for control of the infusion rate. Special tubing must be used to protect from exposure to light which causes decomposition of the nitroglycerin into cyanide.

A is incorrect because intravenous nitroglycerin is only given through an infusion pump for continuous infusion.

B is incorrect because dosing must be adjusted every <u>hour</u> to prevent hypotension, relieve angina, and prevent reflex tachycardia. The infusion is started at 5 mcg/min. Increase by 5 mcg/min every 3-5 min as needed up to 20 mcg/min initially.

D is incorrect because intravenous nitroglycerin is only given through an infusion pump to prevent hypotension and reflex tachycardia.

43. A patient is beginning therapy with diltiazem. Which statement by the patient indicates a need for further instructions by the nurse?

    A. "I can take this medication when I experience angina."
    B. "Food and antacids can alter how the medication is absorbed."
    C. "The long-acting form of the medication can't be crushed."
    D. "The medication can cause drops in blood pressure, so I should be careful when getting out of bed."

Rationale:

Correct answer: A

Diltiazem is a calcium channel blocker given to prevent cardiac muscle contraction and promote muscle relaxation, causing dilation of the coronary arteries. Afterload is also decreased, reducing myocardial oxygen demand. Diltiazem specifically is administered for atrial flutter and atrial fibrillation, not for angina.

B is incorrect because it is a true statement, demonstrating correct patient understanding. Food and antacids do alter the absorption of the drug, and therefore the patient should be instructed not to take this medication with food or antacids such as magnesium hydroxide and aluminum hydroxide.

C is incorrect because this is a true statement, demonstrating correct patient understanding. Extended-release tablets cannot be crushed. They should be taken whole without chewing.

D is incorrect because this is a true statement, demonstrating correct patient understanding. Calcium channel blockers decrease blood pressure and can cause orthostatic hypotension, which poses a risk for falls. This is a safety concern and is important for the nurse to communicate to the patient.

44. A patient is beginning therapy with digoxin PO for heart failure. The nurse educates the patient regarding signs and symptoms of digoxin toxicity which include:

    A. Increased appetite

B. Halos around lights or flickering of lights

C. Low potassium

D. Increased urine output during the day

Rationale:

Correct answer: B

Digoxin is a cardiac glycoside used to treat systolic heart failure and atrial fibrillation. It works by increasing myocardial contractility, enhancing vagal tone, and enhancing conduction through the SA and AV nodes of the heart. This leads to improved cardiac output, decreased heart rate, and increased coronary circulation. Signs of toxicity include bradycardia, dizziness, confusion, and visual disturbances, including halos.

A is incorrect because digoxin toxicity can cause decreased appetite.

C is incorrect because hypokalemia is not a sign of digoxin toxicity. Rather, hypokalemia puts a patient at higher risk for digoxin toxicity.

D is incorrect because digoxin toxicity can cause decreased urine output or excessive urination during the night.

Remember, digoxin has a narrow therapeutic range and requires frequent blood monitoring. The normal range for digoxin is 0.5-2.0 ng/ml in the blood. Anything above

2ng/mL in the blood is considered toxic. The loading dose for digoxin is 0.5 – 0.75 mg PO, and then the maintenance dose is 0.125 – 0.375 mg PO daily until the clinical effect is achieved.

45. A patient has intravenous nesiritide infusing for heart failure. The nurse knows to monitor for which adverse effect?

    A. Dysrhythmia
    B. Increased protein in the urine
    C. Fasting blood glucose 150 mg/dL
    D. Blood pressure 152/95 mm/Hg

Rationale:

Correct answer: A

Nesiritide is a B-type natriuretic peptide that is used to treat patients with heart failure and exhibit difficulty breathing during rest or minimal activity. The intended action of the medication is vasodilation, making it easier for the heart to deliver oxygen through the body. This leads to increased cardiac output, increased urine output, and suppression of the renin-angiotensin system. Adverse effects of nesiritide include hypotension, dysrhythmias, abdominal pain, and headache.

B is incorrect because proteinuria is not an adverse effect of nesiritide.

C is incorrect because hyperglycemia is not an adverse effect of nesiritide. (Normal fasting blood glucose is 60-110 mg/dL.)

D is incorrect because hypertension is not an adverse effect of nesiritide. This medication will actually help with hypertension.

46. A patient is admitted to the emergency room for "racing heart." The healthcare provider orders adenosine to be administered. While administering the adenosine, the nurse initially anticipates which effect?

    A. Increased cardiac output
    B. Asystole
    C. Muscle tetany
    D. Sinus rhythm

    Rationale:

    Correct answer: B

    Adenosine is an unclassified antidysrhythmic that works by slowing conduction through the AV node to convert rapid rhythms such as paroxysmal supraventricular tachycardia (PSVT) back to sinus rhythm. It can only be administered by rapid IV push as the half-life is extremely short. The expected effect is temporary asystole. Common side effects are facial flushing and light-headedness. More serious adverse reactions are worsening dysrhythmia and hypotension.

A is incorrect because the purpose of adenosine

C is incorrect because adenosine does not affect skeletal muscle action.

D is incorrect because adenosine will initially cause asystole and then convert back to sinus rhythm.

47. The nurse is initiating a lidocaine infusion for a patient experiencing frequent premature ventricular contractions (PVCs). Which of the following conditions would warrant a dosage reduction for patient safety?

    A. Tachycardia
    B. Hypertension
    C. Ventricular dysrhythmias
    D. Liver failure

Rationale:

Correct answer: D

Lidocaine is an antidysrhythmic given for ventricular dysrhythmias including frequent PVCs. It functions by preventing dysrhythmia formation in the ventricles.

Lidocaine is metabolized in the liver, so patients with liver failure would require a dosage reduction. Dosage reduction is also recommended for patients with kidney dysfunction.

A is incorrect because tachycardia is not an indication for lidocaine.

B is incorrect because hypertension is not an indication for lidocaine.

C is incorrect because ventricular dysrhythmias are an indication for lidocaine but not for dosage reduction.

48. A patient experiencing chest pain is admitted to the emergency room to rule out MI. The nurse is administering a thrombolytic intravenously. Which of the following would be most concerning to the nurse?

    A. Dizziness
    B. Blood pressure 132/96 mmHg
    C. Slight bleeding at the IV site
    D. Irregular heart rhythm

Rationale:

Correct answer: D

Thrombolytic medications modify coagulation to lyse clots in blood vessels through converting plasminogen to plasmin. This can help restore blood flow to blocked coronary arteries. These medications are nonspecific when given IV, so they can break down clots anywhere in the vasculature, putting the patient at risk for bleeding. Indications include MI, DVT, occluded catheters, PE, and ischemic stroke with acute onset. Thrombolytic medications are contraindicated for use in conjunction with other medications that alter clotting. Patients with irregular heart rates are at an increased risk for further clotting, and a thrombotic medication could cause these clots to circulate throughout the body leading to stroke or MI.

A is incorrect because dizziness is not of great concern during thrombolytic therapy. However, an altered level of consciousness can be a sign of hemorrhagic stroke, so this would need to be investigated further by the nurse.

B is incorrect because the blood pressure is within normal limits. Hypertension would be concerning due to the risk of hemorrhagic stroke.

C is incorrect because some bleeding at the IV site is to be expected when administering a thrombolytic.

49. A patient is beginning treatment with warfarin for atrial fibrillation. Which of the following patient statements is most concerning to the nurse?

A. "I take oxycodone for chronic pain related to fibromyalgia."
B. "I understand that I can still take acetaminophen if I have a headache."
C. "I understand that I should avoid NSAIDs."
D. "I understand that I must eliminate all garlic from my diet."

Rationale:

Correct answer: D

Garlic should not be taken as a daily supplement when the patient is taking warfarin because garlic thins the blood, and this can increase the risk for bleeding. But this patient needs to be educated that a small amount of dietary garlic is still acceptable without putting the patient at a greater risk of bleeding.

A is incorrect because opioids such as oxycodone are safe to take with warfarin.

B is incorrect because acetaminophen and warfarin are not contraindicated for use together. However, chronic use of acetaminophen can increase the risk for bleeding. This patient should be counseled to only take acetaminophen when needed, but not daily.

C is incorrect because NSAIDs and warfarin should not be used together. NSAIDs, or non-steroidal anti-inflammatory drugs, work by decreasing platelet activity to decrease the formation of clots. Any medication that alters clotting will have an additive effect with warfarin, increasing the risk of bleeding.

50. A patient is being sent home with a prescription for enoxaparin. When teaching the patient about the administration of the enoxaparin, which statement should the nurse include?

    A. "We will also need to teach your wife how to give the medication in your arm."
    B. "The medication should be given in the abdomen at least two inches from your navel."
    C. "Take the medication daily at the same time with eight ounces of water."
    D. "Massage the site well after the injection."

Rationale:

Correct answer: B

Enoxaparin is low molecular weight heparin that prevents and treats the formation of clots. It is indicated for patients who have unstable angina, post-surgery, and after MI. It works by interfering with factor X which is necessary for the formation of clots. Enoxaparin must be given in the abdomen at least 2 inches away from the navel as it is better absorbed through the fatty tissue.

A is incorrect because enoxaparin is only administered in the abdomen.

C is incorrect because water is not necessary to take when giving a self-injection of enoxaparin.

D is incorrect because the site must not be massaged as it can cause bruising.

51. A patient received two doses of heparin during a coronary artery bypass grafting procedure. The post-operative nurse notes bright red blood through the dressing. What medication order will the nurse anticipate?

    A. IV vitamin K
    B. IV protamine sulfate
    C. Platelet transfusion
    D. Packed red blood cells

Rationale:

Correct answer: B

Heparin is a natural anticoagulant that is commonly used during coronary artery bypass grafting surgery. It is also used prophylactically to prevent DVT and PE. The antidote for heparin is protamine sulfate 1.0 – 1.5 mg per 100 units of heparin within the last 4 hours. PTT should be monitored 5 to 15 minutes and 2 to 8 hours after protamine sulfate IV is administered.

A is incorrect because vitamin K is not the antidote for heparin. Vitamin K is the antidote for warfarin.

C is incorrect because platelet transfusion will not reverse the action of heparin.

D is incorrect because packed red blood cells will not reverse the action of heparin. Only if the protamine sulfate is not effective in reversing the heparin and the patient loses a significant amount of blood will a transfusion of PRBCs be indicated.

52. The nurse is administering niacin to a patient. Which assessment will be most concerning to the nurse?

    A. Cutaneous flushing

    B. Pale urine

    C. Hypoglycemia

    D. Improvement in gout symptoms

Rationale:

Correct answer: A

Niacin is a B vitamin that is unique in its lipid-lowering capabilities. It works on the effects of lipoproteins in the plasma and is often given in combination with other lipid-lowering medications. Niacin causes flushing, itching, and GI distress. Low-dose aspirin can be taken before niacin to reduce cutaneous flushing.

B is incorrect because an adverse reaction to niacin will produce dark-colored urine. Pale urine is not related to niacin use.

C is incorrect because niacin can cause hyperglycemia, not hypoglycemia.

D is incorrect because niacin does can actually cause gout. The nurse would not be concerned if gout symptoms improved with the use of niacin.

53. A patient is beginning treatment with atorvastatin. Which of the following will the nurse include in the patient education?

   A. "Take the atorvastatin with each meal to reduce the cholesterol absorbed in your small intestine."
   B. "This medication does not necessitate a low-fat diet."
   C. "Report any muscle pain to the healthcare provider immediately."
   D. "You can expect to see improved cholesterol levels within the next 2 weeks."

Rationale:

Correct answer: C

Atorvastatin decreases cholesterol production by the liver, thereby decreasing serum cholesterol levels. Muscle pain can be a sign of rhabdomyolysis, a rare yet serious complication of statin medications. This can lead to renal failure. Other less serious side effects of statins include abdominal pain, rash, and headache.

A is incorrect because atorvastatin should be taken 1 hour before evening meals.

B is incorrect because a low-fat diet is beneficial for reducing serum cholesterol in addition to taking a statin medication.

D is incorrect because therapeutic effects will be revealed by lab tests within 1 to 3 months of initiating statin therapy.

54. A patient is receiving furosemide and hydrochlorothiazide. When lab tests are drawn, the nurse expects to see which results?

  A. Serum potassium 3.2 mEq/L
  B. Total serum calcium 12.7 mg/dL
  C. Serum glucose 55 mg/dL
  D. Serum sodium 151 mEq/L

Rationale:

Correct answer: A

Furosemide, a loop diuretic, and hydrochlorothiazide, a thiazide diuretic, both inhibit the reabsorption of potassium. This would lead to potassium wasting with the fluids that are excreted from the kidneys. Combining these medications would cause decreased potassium level or hypokalemia.

B is incorrect because neither loop nor thiazide diuretics cause hypercalcemia.

C is incorrect because neither loop nor thiazide diuretics cause hypoglycemia. Thiazides can actually cause hyperglycemia.

D is incorrect because both loop and thiazide diuretics prevent sodium from being reabsorbed, leading to hyponatremia.

- Remember: the nurse should instruct the patient that when taking furosemide and hydrochlorothiazide:
  - Don't take at bedtime
  - Monitor weight, I/O
  - Increased intake of potassium-rich foods

55. A patient with diabetes is started on hydrochlorothiazide. When the nurse teaches the patient about HCTZ, which of the following statements should be included?

A. "HCTZ is a safe drug with little concern for complications."
B. "Avoid eating foods that have high levels of potassium."
C. "Take the HCTZ at bedtime so it won't interfere with your diabetes medications."
D. "Be sure to check your blood sugar routinely."

Rationale:

Correct answer: D

HCTZ is a thiazide diuretic that works by preventing the reabsorption of potassium and sodium. An adverse effect of HCTZ is hyperglycemia, which is more pronounced in patients with diabetes.

A is incorrect because the patient needs to be educated about the concerns related to HCTZ: risk for hypokalemia, hyponatremia, hyperglycemia, and fatigue.

B is incorrect because thiazide diuretics can cause hypokalemia, so patients should be encouraged to increase their intake of foods containing potassium such as: white beans, spinach, baked potatoes (with skin), dried apricots, acorn squash, and yogurt. Hypokalemia can cause fatigue, irritability, and hypertension.

C is incorrect because HCTZ is a diuretic that will increase the need to urinate. This can disrupt the sleep-wake cycle, cause night time bed-wetting, and pose a risk for falls when getting up in the middle of the night to go to the bathroom.

56. A patient is to receive packed red blood cells by infusion for the treatment of a gastric hemorrhage. Which of the following is an appropriate nursing action for this patient?

    A. Before the blood transfusion begins, flush IV with normal saline
    B. Before the blood transfusion begins, flush IV with normal D_5W
    C. Check vital signs upon completion of the infusion
    D. Expect mild facial flushing and slightly decreased temperature in response to the transfusion

    Rationale:

    Correct answer: A

    Flush the IV with normal saline before adding blood to the infusion.

    Blood transfusions are high risk and require frequent monitoring and careful preparation. The most appropriate action before transfusing red blood cells is to flush the patient's IV with normal saline.

B is incorrect because blood can only be administered with 0.9 NaCl. The D$_5$W contains glucose, which is incompatible for use when administering blood or blood products.

C is incorrect because vital signs are checked before a blood transfusion is initiated, 15 minutes after initiation, 30 minutes after initiation, and when the transfusion is complete (dependent upon facility policy).

D is incorrect because flushing is a sign of a reaction to the blood. The transfusion should be stopped immediately, and the nurse must change the IV tubing and resume the normal saline infusion. Then, the primary healthcare provider should be notified. Low temperature is not a sign of a reaction to a blood transfusion, but it is also not a common response.

57. The nurse is preparing IV fluids with potassium for several patients. Which of the following would cause the nurse to hold the fluid and call the healthcare provider?

    A. The patient had gastric-bypass surgery yesterday and is experiencing dumping syndrome
    B. Patient being treated for Cushing's Syndrome, with a sodium level of 140 mEq/L
    C. The patient admitted for abdominal pain with a potassium level of 2.7 mEq/L

D. The patient admitted yesterday with deep-partial-thickness burns to the lower abdomen and lower extremities, experiencing dehydration

Rationale:

Correct answer: D.

Burn patients are at risk for hyperkalemia. Although they are at risk for dehydration, Lactated Ringer's solution is the fluid of choice initially. Burn patients need a high-calorie, high-protein, high-carbohydrate diet and may potentially need additional tube feeding to meet dietary needs for adequate healing, even if they are taking in PO food and fluids.

A is incorrect because dumping syndrome is characterized by frequent diarrhea, which causes hypokalemia and metabolic acidosis (potassium and base loss in stool). This patient would benefit from the potassium IV fluid replacement to correct the dehydration and hypokalemia.

B is incorrect because this is a normal serum sodium level and is not contraindicated with potassium. Patients with Cushing's Syndrome are at risk for hypernatremia and hypokalemia. This patient would likely benefit from the potassium fluid replacement.

C is incorrect because this patient has a low serum potassium level and would benefit from a potassium replacement fluid.

58. A patient with hemophilia is admitted to the medical unit. Which of the following does the nurse anticipate to include in the plan of care for this patient?

    A. 5% albumin IV at 12 mL / minute
    B. 2 units packed red blood cells
    C. Activity as tolerated
    D. Fresh frozen plasma

Rationale:

Correct answer: D

Patients with clotting disorders require clotting factors in order to improve the clotting and prevent bleeding. Fresh frozen plasma will increase clotting factor levels. Remember: administration of plasma increases the risk for circulatory overload. Plasma must be administered quickly with a straight IV set, as the coagulation factors may become unstable.

A is incorrect because 5% albumin is a crystalloid for expanding plasma and shifting fluid back into the intravascular space. The hemophilia patient does not need a plasma-volume expander; this patient needs clotting factors, which are not provided by albumin. Albumin is hypertonic, and thus it increases the risk for circulatory volume overload. When indicated (high intracranial pressure, for example), albumin should be started at a rate of 2-3 mL/minute. A rate above 10 mL/min is not safe for the administration of albumin.

B is incorrect because packed red blood cells do not provide the clotting factors. The clotting factors are found in plasma, which has been removed from the PRBCs.

C is incorrect because patients with hemophilia are generally in the hospital for bleeding problems, and bed rest is required.

59. A patient has a crystalloid solution infusing at 150 mL/hr through a subclavian triple lumen catheter for treatment of septic shock. Which of the following assessments is most concerning to the nurse?

    A. Heartrate 58 bpm
    B. Blood pressure 98/52 mmHg
    C. Decreased skin turgor and temperature 102.4 °F (39.1 °C)
    D. Pre-tibial edema and crackles that clear when coughing

Rationale:

Correct answer: D

Crystalloids are administered for fluids and sodium to maintain extravascular and intravascular fluid balance. The most common crystalloids are 0.9% normal saline and Ringer's lactate. Fluid balance, or intake and output, must be monitored to prevent fluid overload. Edema in the lower extremities and crackles are signs of fluid volume overload, which is a complication of crystalloids running at a high hourly flow rate. Even crackles that "clear when coughing" is an early sign that this patient is beginning to retain fluid in the lungs. This is the primary concern.

A is incorrect because crystalloids do not cause bradycardia. The greatest concern when giving a crystalloid (such as normal saline) at a rapid rate is fluid volume overload.

B is incorrect because crystalloids do not cause hypotension. Low blood pressure is not a sign of fluid volume overload.

C is incorrect because a rapid hourly rate of crystalloid infusion is more likely to cause edema as a sign of fluid volume overload. Decreased skin turgor is an assessment the nurse would expect to find with dehydration. An elevated temperature is expected in a patient experiencing septic shock. The fluids are being given to maintain fluid balance, not reduce the temperature.

Medications such as acetaminophen will reduce the temperature, and antibiotics will be given to treat the infection causing the septicemia.

60. A patient taking methimazole calls the clinic nurse to report that she is running low on the medication and the pharmacy has it on backorder. What is the appropriate response by the nurse?

    A. "You can take the other brand that is available until your prescription is available."

    B. "Stop the medication when you run out, and wait until your prescription is available."

    C. "Split the medication in half so you will have more."

    D. "I will notify the healthcare provider to determine if the brand can be safely switched."

Rationale:

Correct answer: D

Methimazole is an antithyroid medication that inhibits the synthesis of thyroid hormone by the thyroid gland. Thyroid levels must be monitored through blood tests. When medication brands are switched, the thyroid hormones can be affected. The healthcare provider should be notified when brands are switched so appropriate monitoring can be performed.

A is incorrect because the healthcare provider should be contacted so an appropriate brand can be chosen and appropriate blood monitoring performed.

B is incorrect because stopping the medication could cause symptoms of hyperthyroidism to return. Remember that signs of hyperthyroidism include: hyperactivity, sensitivity to heat, rest and sleep deprivation, weight loss, diarrhea, exophthalmos, frequent mood swings, and tachycardia.

C is incorrect because dosage should not be altered without monitoring performed. It is not within the nurse's scope of practice to change a medication dosage. Remember: when giving methimazole, teach the client to take this medication with meals and to report fever or sore throat to the health care provider.

61. A 68-year-old patient is starting levothyroxine treatment. From the nurse's knowledge, which of the following is true regarding levothyroxine?

    A. Dosage is approximately 25% lower than younger adults
    B. This medication may cause sleepiness
    C. Dysrhythmias are common when taking this medication
    D. Dosing is dietary iodine-dependent

Rationale:

Correct answer: A

Thyroid replacement hormones work in the same way as endogenous thyroid hormones to regulate metabolic rate, oxygen consumption, temperature, and cellular growth. For older adults (over the age of 60), the dosage is 25% lower.

B is incorrect because levothyroxine has the same effects as thyroid hormone and can cause insomnia, nervousness, tremors, tachycardia, and palpitations.

C is incorrect because dysrhythmias are an adverse reaction to levothyroxine and should be reported to the health care provider.

D is incorrect because the iodine in the diet has no impact on hormone replacement needs.

62. A patient has lispro ordered for treatment of type 1 diabetes mellitus. The nurse knows the best time to administer this type of insulin is:

   A. 5 to 15 minutes prior to a meal
   B. 30 minutes prior to a meal
   C. 60 minutes after a meal
   D. Lispro should be given IV once daily, in the evening

Rationale:

Correct answer: A

Lispro is a rapid-acting insulin. This medication reduces blood glucose levels by increasing glucose transport across cell membranes; it enhances the conversion of glucose to glycogen. The onset of action is 5 to 15 minutes after administration, so the optimal time for administration is 5 to 15 minutes prior to a meal. This will enable the medication to begin working when the patient begins eating. The nurse should not administer a rapid-acting insulin if a meal is going to be delayed, as this can cause hypoglycemia.

B is incorrect because the onset of lispro is 5 to 15 minutes, so the administration of this medication 30 minutes prior to a meal can cause hypoglycemia. Signs of hypoglycemia include trembling and weakness.

C is incorrect because this can cause hyperglycemia. The patient needs his insulin before the meal begins. The peak effect of lispro will be seen at 0.5 2 hours after administration. The duration of action is 3 to 6 hours.

D is incorrect because the timing of administration of any rapid-acting insulin in relation to meals is essential to prevent hypoglycemia. Regular insulin is the only type that can be given IV. All others, including lispro, are given subcutaneously.

63. A 28-year-old patient has recently been diagnosed with type 2 diabetes. Which statement is important for the nurse to include when teaching this patient about the new diagnosis?

    A. "Type 2 diabetes will not require insulin injections."
    B. "You will not have to check your blood sugar because insulin injections are not part of your treatment plan."
    C. "Your pancreas still has beta cells functioning, even though you have type 2 diabetes."
    D. "Type 2 diabetes is more common in childhood and can be treated with diet and exercise."

Rationale:

Correct answer: C

Type 2 diabetes is a condition of insulin resistance due to increased subcutaneous fat in the body. The pancreas still functions with beta cells secreting insulin, but the cells cannot respond to the insulin. Therefore blood glucose levels become increased.

A is incorrect because some patients with type 2 diabetes require insulin injections in addition to oral medications if the oral hypoglycemic agents are not effective at controlling blood glucose levels. The nurse should avoid giving false reassurance. Common oral medications for the control of type 1 diabetes include sulfonylureas, biguanides, alpha-glucosidase inhibitors, and incretin mimetics.

B is incorrect because regardless of the type of diabetes, the blood sugar still needs to be checked routinely.

D is incorrect because type 1 diabetes is more common in childhood. Type 2 is treated with a combination of diet, exercise, and oral medications. Insulin may be indicated.

- Remember the risk factors for type 2 diabetes are:
  - Age over 45
  - Obesity (more than 20% above ideal body weight)
  - Parents or siblings with type 2 diabetes
  - Hypertension
  - High triglyceride levels (greater than 250 mg/dL)
  - History of gestational diabetes
  - Race: African American, Hispanic American, Native American, Asian American
  - Inactive lifestyle

64. The nurse is monitoring a patient who has been taking oral antidiabetic medications for several months. The best

way to identify therapeutic response to oral antidiabetic medications is which of the following?

A. Fewer occurrences of diabetic ketoacidosis (DKA)
B. 5-pound weight loss
C. Glycosylated hemoglobin less than 6%
D. Blood glucose 100 mg/dL

Rationale:

Correct answer: C

Glycosylated hemoglobin is a measurement also known as Hemoglobin A1C. It is used to monitor blood sugar over a 3-month time period, or the typical life span of a red blood cell. This is the most accurate way to measure the effectiveness of oral antidiabetic medications. This test does not require fasting. Normal is 4 to 6%.

A is incorrect because DKA occurs most commonly in type 1 diabetes, for which oral antidiabetics are not used. If a patient has even one episode of DKA, this is a great concern and should be reported to the health care provider.

- Signs of DKA:
  - Blood glucose 300-800 mg/dL
  - Headache, drowsiness, weakness, stupor, coma
  - Warm, dry skin

- Dry mucous membranes (dehydration)
- Polyuria (progressing to oliguria), polydipsia, polyphagia
- Kussmaul's respirations
- Fruity odor to the breath

B is incorrect because weight loss is not an accurate measurement of therapeutic response to oral antidiabetic medications.

D is incorrect because glucose level only shows current blood glucose level. Many factors can affect a one-time blood glucose measurement, such as the time of the last meal, recent medications taken, and stress.

65. A patient is scheduled for computed tomography (CT) with contrast. The patient takes metformin for type 2 diabetes. What is the most appropriate action by the nurse?

    A. Proceed with CT
    B. Notify the radiology department of the patient's medication
    C. Hold the metformin for 24 hours before the CT is scheduled and for 48 hours following the CT
    D. Hold the metformin for 2 days prior to the CT

Rationale:

Correct answer: C

Metformin is an oral biguanide anti-diabetic that inhibits glucose production by the liver and increases peripheral tissue sensitivity to insulin. Iodine contrast media and metformin are both excreted by the kidneys, but the kidneys are unable to excrete both of these products at the same time. This can lead to lactic acidosis and kidney damage. It is important that metformin be held for 24 hours before CT with contrast and for 48 hours afterward to prevent this reaction.

A is incorrect because this patient cannot have their CT with contrast unless the metformin has been held. Metformin could cause renal failure after the CT.

B is incorrect because although the radiology department should be notified of the patient's medication, it is more important for the nurse to hold the medication and postpone the CT procedure. Answer choice C represents the safer nursing action.

D is incorrect because metformin only needs to be held for 24 hours before CT, not 48.

66. A patient's blood glucose has just been checked, and the result is 42 mg/dL. The patient is alert but trembling and states, "I feel like my head is cloudy." The nurse re-checks

blood glucose with the same result. What is the most appropriate action by the nurse?

A. Have the patient eat two packets of sugar
B. Administer oral glucose
C. Administer IV push 50% dextrose
D. Administer lispro

Rationale:

Correct answer: B

This patient is exhibiting signs of hypoglycemia. Oral glucose is administered to counteract hypoglycemia. This patient is speaking and is alert. Oral glucose is appropriate to raise his blood sugar until a meal is delivered. Oral glucose is only indicated for patients who are awake enough to swallow and do not have the risk of aspiration.

A is incorrect because table sugar will not give an accurate amount of glucose to raise blood sugar and may cause hyperglycemia.

C is incorrect because IV glucose is indicated when the patient is unresponsive or too drowsy to swallow oral glucose.

D is incorrect because lispro insulin will decrease the patient's blood sugar even further.

67. The nurse administers prednisone to a patient experiencing an exacerbation of psoriasis. Which of the following statements is appropriate for the nurse to include when discussing the medication with the patient?

    A. "We will draw blood within a week to check for increased lymphocyte count."

    B. "We will watch for this medication to decreased inflammation and skin scales."

    C. "Although this medication does have numerous side effects, you are not likely to get an infection while taking prednisone."

    D. A decrease in Cushing's characteristics

Rationale:

Correct answer: B

Prednisone is a corticosteroid that modifies enzyme activity in the synthesis of proteins. The main effect is inhibiting inflammatory and immune responses. Psoriasis is an auto-immune skin condition that can be treated with prednisone to reduce dry skin patches, itching, burning, and swollen/stiff joints.

A is incorrect because prednisone does not increase lymphocyte levels.

C is incorrect because prednisone can increase susceptibility to infection, and the patient needs to be taught to monitor for signs of infection. Infections may produce few symptoms due to the immune-suppressant activity of the prednisone.

D is incorrect because prednisone can actually cause Cushing's characteristics.

68. A patient has been on long-term corticosteroid therapy. Which of the following characteristics would alert the nurse to possible Cushing's syndrome?

   A. Weight loss and serum sodium 132 mg/dL
   B. Moon face and buffalo hump
   C. Hypotension and bronze skin
   D. Hair thickening

Rationale:

Correct answer: B

A common adverse effect in long-term treatment with corticosteroids is a moon face or hyperadrenocorticism. The face appears round, full, or puffy, and fat builds between the shoulders due to prolonged periods of high levels of cortisol released from the adrenal glands. Other symptoms include mood swings, trunk obesity, blood sugar imbalance, and masculinization in females.

A is incorrect because weight loss and hyponatremia are not symptoms of Cushing's syndrome. These are both signs of Addison's Disease (the opposite of Cushing's). Other Addison's signs: hypotension, hypoglycemia, hyperkalemia, and hyperpigmentation.

C is incorrect because hypotension and bronze skin are both signs of Addison's Disease.

D is incorrect because hair thickening is not a symptom of Cushing's syndrome.

69. A patient with type 2 diabetes and peripheral vascular disease has ciprofloxacin ordered before abdominal surgery in the morning. Sepsis is not present, WBC count is 7800/mm³, and their temperature is 98.6°F (37°C). The nurse knows the purpose for this medication is:

    A. To improve circulation during the procedure
    B. To provide prophylactic therapy
    C. To treat superinfection
    D. To reduce resistant organisms

Rationale:

Correct answer: B

Prophylactic antibiotic therapy is frequently used before surgery to prevent an infection. The risk for infection is higher with abdominal surgery than with other types of surgery, so prophylactic antibiotic therapy is very useful in preventing infection. The risk for infection related to surgery is increased in patients with diabetes, corticosteroid use, obesity, and malnutrition.

A is incorrect because the patient does not need improved circulation during the abdominal surgery. Ciprofloxacin is a fluoroquinolone antibiotic, which will not directly impact circulation.

C is incorrect because there is no superinfection present. Signs of superinfection: fever, diarrhea, glossitis, black hairy tongue, mucous membrane lesions, and vaginal itching/discharge.

D is incorrect because resistant organisms are not reduced with prophylactic antibiotics. The following antibiotics are examples of those used as a "last resort" when treating resistant organisms: amikacin, amphotericin B, polymyxin, and vancomycin.

70. A 17-year-old male takes tetracycline for severe acne. The nurse teaches the patient about precautions with the drug. Which of the following is most important for the nurse to convey?

   A. If improvement is not noted within 2 weeks, the patient should stop taking the tetracycline and call the health care provider
   B. Take the medication with aluminum hydroxide and magnesium trisilicate because GI distress is common

C. Use sunscreen and avoid direct sunlight exposure

D. Teeth should be checked for color changes

Rationale:

Correct answer: C

Tetracycline antibiotics work by preventing bacterial protein synthesis. A common adverse effect of tetracycline is photosensitivity, so patients taking the medication should avoid exposure to sunlight or use sunscreen to prevent rash. The nurse can also teach the patient to wear long-sleeves and a hat when outside.

A is incorrect because tetracycline may take several weeks to months to notice visible results. Therapeutic levels of the medication need to be maintained to prevent further acne from occurring.

B is incorrect because magnesium-containing antacid compounds will affect the absorption of the tetracycline. If stomach upset occurs with tetracycline, the nurse should instruct the patient to take the medication with food (not milk.)

D is incorrect because tetracycline can cause tooth discoloration in deciduous teeth. This is mostly a concern for pregnant women and children under age eight.

71. A nurse receives an accidental needle-stick when caring for a patient who is HIV+. Which drug is recommended for occupational HIV exposure?

   A. Didanosine
   B. Lamivudine and enfuvirtide
   C. Emtricitabine and tenofovir
   D. Acyclovir

Rationale:

Correct answer: C

Emtricitabine and tenofovir are recommended for occupational exposure to HIV.

A is incorrect because didanosine is used in patients with HIV who experience bone marrow suppression. This medication should be chewed or crushed, and liver and renal studies should be monitored.

B is incorrect because lamivudine is indicated for hepatitis B, and enfuvirtide is used for HIV infection combined with another antiretroviral medication.

D is incorrect because acyclovir is used to treat herpes simplex type 1 and type 2, herpes zoster, and chickenpox.

72. A nurse is preparing to administer oral methylcellulose to a patient. The nurse knows a major concern with this medication is:

A. Dehydration
B. Tarry stools
C. Renal calculi
D. Esophageal obstruction

Rationale:

Correct answer: D

Methylcellulose is a laxative that forms bulk and attracts water to be absorbed into the stool, which stimulates intestinal peristalsis. It comes in powder form, which must be mixed with at least eight ounces of liquid. It can congeal and harden, so the medication must be taken immediately, or it can form an esophageal obstruction.

A is incorrect because the laxative attracts excess fluid for stool to add bulk. The effect is more water stool that is easier to pass. This medication may also be used to treat irritable bowel syndrome.

B is incorrect because tarry stools are indicative of a GI bleed which is not an adverse effect of methylcellulose.

C is incorrect because methylcellulose does not cause renal calculi. Side effects include gas and abdominal cramping.

73. A patient was prescribed scopolamine transdermal patches for an upcoming ocean cruise. Which instruction by the nurse is most appropriate?

    A. "Put the patch on 24 hours before traveling."
    B. "Put the patch on 4 hours before traveling."
    C. "Put the patch on the shoulder."
    D. "Put the patch on your temple above the ear."

Rationale:

Correct answer: B

Scopolamine is an anticholinergic used for motion sickness and to reduce secretions prior to surgery. It is placed on the hairless area posterior to the ear at least 4 hours before travel. Scopalamine is contraindicated in patients with angle-closure glaucoma and pyloric obstruction. Side effects include drowsiness, confusion, and disorientation. This medication should be used cautiously with the elderly.

A is incorrect because the patch should be placed 4 hours before traveling for effectiveness.

C is incorrect because the patch should be placed behind the ear. The patch should be replaced every 3 days.

D is incorrect because the patch should be placed behind the ear.

74. A 40-year-old patient is to receive his first chemotherapy treatment for skin cancer. The chemotherapy nurse knows the best timing for his intravenous antiemetic medication is:

    A. 4 hours before initiating chemotherapy
    B. 30 to 60 minutes before initiating chemotherapy
    C. Simultaneous with chemotherapy initiation
    D. When nausea occurs

Rationale:

Correct answer: B

For the best prevention of nausea associated with chemotherapy, the optimal time to administer an antiemetic is 30 to 60 minutes before initiation. Antiemetics such as ondansetron, lorazepam, and metoclopramide are commonly used to prevent chemotherapy-induced nausea.

A is incorrect because the medication will not be as effective after 4 hours.

C is incorrect because nausea will most likely begin to occur before the antiemetic medication becomes effective.

D is incorrect because waiting until nausea occurs will cause greater patient discomfort.

- Remember: the nurse can teach the patient the following measures to help manage nausea related to chemotherapy:

    o Stay hydrated

    o Practice good mouth care

    o Eat small meals

    o Avoid strong smells and spicy foods

75. A patient who is undergoing chemotherapy tells the nurse he learned about phosphorated carbohydrate solution on the Internet as an anti-nausea remedy. When he asks if the drug would help him, what is the best answer by the nurse?

    A. "This could be good for you. Let's talk to the healthcare provider."
    B. "This drug is only used when other drugs have been ineffective."
    C. "This drug interacts dangerously with many chemotherapy medications."
    D. "This drug may not help severe nausea from chemotherapy."

Rationale:

Correct answer: D

Phosphorated carbohydrate solution acts directly on the walls of the GI tract to reduce cramping and control mild nausea and vomiting. It is not sufficient for severe nausea related to chemotherapy.

A is incorrect because it gives the patient false hope. This drug is not sufficient for chemotherapy-induced nausea.

B is incorrect because this medication is only used for mild nausea and vomiting. Lorazepam and metoclopramide are generally more effective in managing chemotherapy-induced nausea.

C is incorrect because while this drug is ineffective for severe nausea and vomiting with chemotherapy, it does not actually pose a risk for dangerous interaction.

Select All That Apply

76. A patient just admitted for chest pain has new medication orders written by the healthcare provider. Which orders will need to be clarified? Select all that apply.

    A. Metformin 500 mg PO twice a day
    B. Sitagliptin 50 mg daily
    C. Simvastatin 20 mg PO every night

D. Irbesartan 300 mg PO once daily

E. Docusate PRN constipation

Rationale:

Correct answer: B, E

Sitagliptin 50 mg daily is missing the route of administration. he healthcare provider must be contacted in order to clarify the route.

Docusate PRN constipation is missing the dosage as well as the route of administration. The healthcare provider must be contacted in order to clarify dosage and route.

All other choices have the medication name, dosage, route, and frequency ordered.

77. The nurse enters a patient's room to administer a scheduled antibiotic on the night shift. The patient states, "I took that already. I don't want to take it again." In order to maintain patient safety, which action should the nurse take? Select all that apply.

    A. Review the chart for medication administration documentation

    B. Contact the pharmacy to see if the medication was delivered

    C. Give the antibiotic dose as scheduled

    D. Notify the healthcare provider

E. Skip the dose and reschedule the next scheduled dose

Rationale:

Correct answer: A, B

Documentation should always be reviewed when medication administration is in question. If it wasn't documented, it wasn't done. Asking the patient about whether or not a medication was previously taken is not always accurate, especially when a patient has multiple medications. Contacting the pharmacy to verify the medication was requested or withdrawn from the medication dispensation machine is always a valid option as medications are typically tracked through a computer system. Another appropriate action would be to contact the nurse who cared for the patient during the previous shift to see if the medication was administered and documentation was missed.

C is incorrect because the medication should not be administered until the nurse determines if the dose has already been given. Some antibiotics are nephrotoxic and cause kidney damage when taken in high doses.

D is incorrect because there is no need to contact the healthcare provider at this time.

E is incorrect because it is crucial to maintain blood levels of antibiotics in order to clear infections. Microorganisms can become resistant to antibiotics when sufficient levels are not maintained.

78. Morphine by the intravenous route is ordered for a post-surgical patient. When educating the patient and family about the medication, which of the following common adverse effects does the nurse inform them can occur with the medication? Select all that apply.

    A. Diarrhea
    B. Constipation
    C. Pruritus
    D. Urinary frequency
    E. Nausea

Rationale:

Correct answer: B, C, E

Morphine is an opioid that slows gastrointestinal tract motility causing constipation and nausea. Morphine can also cause histamine release, which mimics an allergic response, leading to itching. Morphine can also cause drowsiness, sedation, lightheadedness, dizziness, and sweating. Adverse reactions such as seizures, chest pain, or hives should be reported to the health care provider immediately.

A is incorrect because morphine slows gastrointestinal tract motility which leads to constipation.

D is incorrect because morphine causes urinary retention and decreased frequency of urination.

79. A patient is recovering from a major abdominal surgical procedure in the post-anesthesia care unit. The nurse is monitoring for malignant hyperthermia, which is characterized by elevated body temperature as well as which of the following? <u>Select all that apply.</u>

    A. Respirations eight breaths / minute
    B. Respirations 24 breaths / minute
    C. Heartrate 122 BMP
    D. Seizure
    E. Muscle rigidity

Rationale:

Correct answer: B, C, E

Malignant hyperthermia is an uncommon, potentially fatal adverse metabolic reaction to anesthesia. It is genetic in nature and is experienced more often by children, adolescents, and patients with muscular or skeletal abnormalities. It is characterized by elevated body temperature, tachypnea, tachycardia, and muscle rigidity and must be treated with dantrolene, a skeletal muscle relaxant. Cardiac and respiratory supportive care must also be provided.

A is incorrect because malignant hyperthermia is characterized by tachypnea (rapid breathing).

D is incorrect because it is not a characteristic of malignant hyperthermia.

80. A patient has a benzodiazepine ordered as a sedative-hypnotic drug for sleep. Which of the following considerations does the nurse need to remember when administering this medication? Select all that apply.

   A. These medications are for the long-term management of sleeplessness
   B. These medications can be combined with other CNS depressants for sleeplessness
   C. The medication should be administered 1 hour before bedtime
   D. The medication is the first choice for the treatment of sleeplessness
   E. Morning-after drowsiness should be evaluated after the medication is taken

   Rationale:

Correct answer: C, E

Benzodiazepines administered as sedative-hypnotics for sleep are useful for short-term treatment of sleeplessness. These medications shorten the time it takes to fall asleep, so they should be given approximately 1 hour before bedtime. However, they increase light sleep, causing a possibility for drowsiness the morning after taking them.

A is incorrect because these medications are indicated for short-term usage.

B is incorrect because they work synergistically with other CNS depressants, leading to potential adverse reactions such as decreased respiratory rate and lethargy. Alcohol should also be avoided when taking benzodiazepines.

D is incorrect because these medications can cause dependence as well as rebound sleeplessness. Prior to initiating pharmacologic measures for sleep problems, the nurse should instruct the patient to get adequate exercise, ensure a quiet, dark place for sleeping, and eliminate stimulants such as caffeine from the diet.

81. The nurse on the medical unit is preparing to administer carbamazepine to a patient. Which guidelines will the nurse follow? Select all that apply.

    A. Monitor for drowsiness
    B. Stop the medications if seizure activity stops

C. Administer the medication daily at the same time

D. Ensure the patient takes the medication on an empty stomach

E. Notify the healthcare provider if the patient cannot take the medication

Rationale:

Correct answer: A, C, E

Antiepileptic drugs are commonly used for the control and prevention of seizure activity. Common side effects of carbamazepine include nausea and vomiting, as well as dizziness, drowsiness, diplopia, and ataxia. Because of the CNS effects of the medication, the patient's level of consciousness should be monitored. Constant levels of the medications must be maintained in order to prevent seizure activity, so they should be administered at the same time every day. If the patient is unable to take the medication due to GI effects, the healthcare provider must be notified in order to administer the medication by a different route.

B is incorrect because abrupt discontinuation of the medication can lead to seizure activity.

D is incorrect because of the potential for GI upset with this class of medications. Carbamazepine should be taken with food.

82. A patient is taking diltiazem for atrial fibrillation. Which of the following effects does the nurse expect to find when assessing the patient? Select all that apply.

   A. Reduced blood pressure
   B. Decreased heart rate
   C. Increased ectopic beats
   D. Increased cardiac output
   E. Decreased edema

Rationale:

Correct answer: A, B, D

Diltiazem is a calcium channel blocker commonly given for atrial fibrillation. It works by preventing the flow of calcium through the NA-K channel, thereby decreasing stimulation of the conduction system of the heart. This will lead to decreased heart rate, decreased blood pressure, and increased cardiac output due to less systemic vascular resistance.

C is incorrect because decreased ectopic beats will be seen with calcium channel blockers.

E is incorrect because calcium channel blockers do not have a direct effect on edema. Diuretics, such as furosemide, will lead to decreased edema.

83. The nurse is preparing to initiate a norepinephrine infusion for a patient in shock. Which nursing interventions will the nurse include? <u>Select all that apply.</u>

    A. Monitor for increased blood pressure

    B. Protect the medication from bright light

    C. Infuse with normal saline

    D. Expect decreased heart rate

    E. Increased stroke volume

Rationale:

Correct answer: A, B

Norepinephrine works by stimulating alpha-1 receptors to cause vasoconstriction and increased blood pressure and beta-1 receptors to increase heart rate, blood pressure, and cardiac output. Norepinephrine must be kept from exposure to bright light.

C is incorrect because norepinephrine should be infused with a dextrose solution.

D is incorrect because norepinephrine will cause an increase in heart rate.

E is incorrect because norepinephrine will have no effect on the stroke volume of the heart.

84. A patient diagnosed with Alzheimer's disease is admitted to the medical unit for toxic levels of donepezil. Which of the following adverse effects would the nurse expect to find? <u>Select all that apply.</u>

    A. Constipation

    B. GI upset

    C. Drowsiness

    D. Dizziness

    E. Blurred vision

Rationale:

Correct answer: B, C, D

Donepezil is a cholinesterase inhibitor used to treat mild or moderate Alzheimer's disease. Adverse effects include GI upset, drowsiness, dizziness, diarrhea, loss of appetite, and muscle cramps.

A is incorrect because the medication can cause diarrhea, not constipation.

E is incorrect because the medication does not cause visual disturbances.

85. A patient prescribed isosorbide dinitrate for angina symptoms is admitted to the medical unit for observation. When the nurse reviews his medication reconciliation and

history, which of the following is most concerning? Select all that apply.

A. The patient drinks a glass of grapefruit juice each morning
B. The patient takes thyroid replacement hormone
C. The patient takes tadalafil
D. The patient takes metformin
E. The patient takes carvedilol

Rationale:

Correct answer: C, E

Isosorbide dinitrate is a nitrate prescribed for angina that causes vasodilation and smooth muscle relaxation. Tadalafil and carvedilol will cause further vasodilation that can lead to severe hypotension when combined with nitrate medication.

A is incorrect because grapefruit juice does not interact with isosorbide dinitrate.

B is incorrect because there is no interaction between nitrates and thyroid replacement hormone.

D is incorrect because there is no interaction between nitrates and metformin.

86. Intravenous phosphodiesterase inhibitor is administered to a patient with heart failure. The nurse knows

therapeutic effects of this treatment include: <u>Select all that apply.</u>

- A. Increased contractility
- B. Vasodilation
- C. Decreased heart rate
- D. Increased blood pressure
- E. Increased heart rate

Rationale:

Correct answer: A, B, E

Phosphodiesterase inhibitors (such as milrinone) are inotropic drugs that inhibit phosphodiesterase found in the heart and vascular smooth muscles. This medication causes positive inotrope and vasodilation effects. The effects include increased contractility, vasodilation, and increased heart rate. Adverse effects include hypokalemia and dysrhythmias.

C is incorrect because phosphodiesterase inhibitors cause increased heart rate.

D is incorrect because phosphodiesterase inhibitors cause decreased blood pressure.

87. A patient diagnosed with heart failure is starting treatment with metoprolol. The nurse expects to see

which of the following cardiovascular effects? <u>Select all that apply.</u>

A. Increased heart rate

B. Increased contractility

C. Delayed conduction through the AV node

D. Decreased heart rate

E. Decreased automaticity

Rationale:

Correct answer: C, D, E

Metoprolol is a beta-blocker that causes delayed conduction through the AV node, decreased heart rate, and decreased automaticity as therapeutic effects in heart failure. It works by blocking the stimulation of the beta-1 receptors in the heart.

A is incorrect because beta-blockers do not cause increased heart rate. The nurse would expect the metoprolol to decrease the heart rate, and the medication should be withheld if the heart rate is below 60 bpm.

B is incorrect because beta-blockers do not cause increased contractility.

88. A patient has been prescribed amiodarone for atrial fibrillation. When teaching the patient regarding

antidysrhythmic medications, which statements are correct? Select all that apply.

A. "If your stomach gets upset, take an antacid with the medication."
B. "Extended-release capsules cannot be chewed."
C. "If you gain 5 or more pounds within a week, notify the healthcare provider at your next scheduled appointment."
D. "Stop taking the medication and notify the healthcare provider if you notice uncomfortable side effects."
E. "If your stomach gets upset, take the medication with a meal."

Rationale:

Correct answer: B, E

Antidysrhythmic medications are taken to regulate heart rate and rhythm. If an extended-release form is taken, the pill cannot be cut, crushed, or chewed. If stomach upset occurs, this medication can be taken with food.

A is incorrect because antacids can alter the absorption of the antidysrhythmic.

C is incorrect because a weight gain of 5 pounds in a week warrants immediate notification of the healthcare provider as it is indicative of heart failure. Some fluid retention and weight gain may be acceptable with heart failure, but more than 2 lbs daily, or 5 lbs in a week, is a concern.

D is incorrect because discontinuation of an antidysrhythmic can cause reflex tachycardia, dysrhythmias, and hypotension.

89. A patient is taking warfarin for atrial fibrillation. Which principles regarding warfarin therapy does the nurse follow? <u>Select all that apply.</u>

    A. Teach the patient how to administer the medication subcutaneously

    B. Take the warfarin at the same time daily

    C. Look for unusual bleeding or bruising

    D. Monitor INR for target 2.0 to 3.5

    E. Monitor PTT for target 1.5 to 2.5 times control value

Rationale:

Correct answer: B, C, D

Warfarin inhibits the synthesis of vitamin K, thereby inhibiting the production of several clotting factors normally made in the liver. It is a PO medication that must be taken at the same time daily to maintain blood levels. Because it interferes with clotting factors, the patient must watch for unusual bleeding or bruising, which could indicate injury or internal hemorrhaging. The prothrombin time and internationalized normalized ratio (PT/INR) should be monitored. The INR therapeutic range while taking warfarin is 2.0 to 3.5.

A is incorrect because warfarin is a PO medication.

E is incorrect because PTT is monitored when heparin is being administered, not warfarin.

90. A 75-year-old patient is being discharged with a new prescription for furosemide after heart failure exacerbation. When providing discharge instructions, which of the following does the nurse provide? <u>Select all that apply.</u>

    A. "Take the furosemide every morning at the same time."

    B. "Only take the furosemide if you notice your feet swelling."

    C. "Stand up slowly to prevent dizziness."

    D. "Drink twelve glasses of water daily."

    E. "Avoid eating foods that have high levels of potassium."

    F. "If you experience weakness or increased dizziness, notify your healthcare provider immediately."

Rationale:

Correct answer: A, C, F

Furosemide is a loop diuretic that must be taken at the same time daily to rid the body of excess fluids. Due to fluid loss, it is important to stand up slowly to prevent orthostatic hypotension, which can increase the risk for and falls. Due to the potential for hypokalemia, the healthcare provider should be notified of muscle weakness, as this may be a sign of hypokalemia which may require additional cardiac monitoring or potassium supplementation. Furosemide can also cause hyperglycemia.

B is incorrect because the furosemide should be taken daily whether or not swelling is present.

D is incorrect because furosemide is taken for diuresis, and additional fluids can contribute to fluid retention and edema. I&O should be monitored, and the patient should be instructed not to take the medication at night.

E is incorrect because furosemide is a potassium-wasting diuretic. Patients taking this medication should be instructed to consume foods high in potassium to prevent hypokalemia.

91. A patient in the intensive care unit is receiving an infusion of IV fluids with potassium chloride for hypokalemia.

Which of the following interventions does the nurse provide for this patient? <u>Select all that apply.</u>

A. Slow IV gravity bolus administration

B. Administer potassium no faster than 20 mEq/hr

C. Place the patient on a monitor and observe the cardiac rhythm

D. Use an infusion pump for the potassium

E. Administer potassium fast by IV push

Rationale:

Correct answer: B, C, D

Potassium is commonly given in IV fluid as well as in piggybacks to boost potassium levels in those who are hypokalemic. The fluids and piggybacks must always be infused using an IV pump and no faster than 20 mEq/hr. The patient must also be on a cardiac monitor to monitor heart rhythm because potassium levels affect the heart rhythm. Potassium is needed for cell growth and normal functioning of cardiac, skeletal, and smooth muscles.

A is incorrect because potassium is never given by IV bolus without the use of an infusion pump.

E is incorrect because potassium is never given by IV push without the use of an infusion pump. Cardiac complications can occur.

92. A patient has a new prescription for levothyroxine. The nurse instructs the patient to notify the healthcare provider if which of the following adverse effects are noticed? Select all that apply.

    A. Palpitations
    B. Weight gain
    C. Angina
    D. Fatigue
    E. Intolerance to cold

Rationale:

Correct answer: A, C

Levothyroxine and other thyroid hormone replacement therapies work to replace the normal hormones in a hypothyroid patient. When levels get too high, the patient experiences symptoms of hyperthyroidism, which include palpitations, angina, sweating, and nervousness. The healthcare provider should be notified if these symptoms occur so the dosing can be altered.

B is incorrect because weight gain is not an adverse effect of thyroid hormone replacement therapy. Weight gain and obesity are symptoms of hypothyroidism.

D is incorrect because fatigue is not an adverse effect of thyroid hormone replacement therapy. Levothyroxine is more likely to give the patient a boost of energy.

E is incorrect because cold intolerance is not an adverse effect of thyroid hormone replacement therapy. Hypothyroid patients commonly experience sensitivity to cold, while hyperthyroid patients experience heat sensitivity.

93. A patient has come to the healthcare provider's office to have a lab drawn to monitor thyroid hormone replacement therapy effectiveness. Which of the following does the nurse anticipate drawing? <u>Select all that apply.</u>

    A. Serum TSH
    B. BUN
    C. CBC
    D. Free thyroid hormone level
    E. Serum iodine level

Rationale:

Correct answer: A, D

Routine blood tests must be checked in order to monitor the effectiveness of thyroid hormone replacement therapy. These tests include serum TSH (thyroid-stimulating hormone) and free thyroid hormone levels. These tests will demonstrate how effective the thyroid is functioning with the assistance of thyroid hormone replacement therapy. TSH is generally elevated in hypothyroid patients (because the thyroid is not making enough thyroid hormone). So a normal TSH level would indicate improvement with this medication.

B is incorrect because BUN (blood urea nitrogen) demonstrates kidney function.

C is incorrect because CBC does not indicate thyroid function.

E is incorrect because although it is related to thyroid function, it does not demonstrate the effectiveness of thyroid hormone replacement therapy.

94. A patient was recently diagnosed with type 2 diabetes, for which he is taking metformin. The nurse is preparing to discuss the potential adverse effects of metformin with the patient. Which of the following will the nurse include? Select all that apply.

    A. Abdominal bloating
    B. Nausea
    C. Diarrhea
    D. Headache
    E. Weight gain

Rationale:

Correct answer: A, B, C

Metformin is an oral biguanide anti-diabetic that inhibits glucose production by the liver and increases peripheral tissue sensitivity to insulin. Potential adverse effects of metformin include abdominal bloating, nausea, and diarrhea. Metformin is not given to patients with renal impairment. Alcohol should be avoided. This medication can cause lactic acidosis.

D is incorrect because a headache is not an adverse effect of metformin.

E is incorrect because weight gain is not an adverse effect of metformin.

95. A patient has been on long-term corticosteroid therapy for 2 years. The nurse is aware that lab results will be monitored for which of the following adverse effects? Select all that apply.

   A. Potassium 5.8 mEq/L
   B. Potassium 3.2 mEq/L
   C. Total serum calcium 7.1 mg/dL
   D. Magnesium 1.1 mEq/L
   E. Blood glucose 160 mg/dL
   F. Hematocrit 48%

Rationale:

Correct answer: B, C, E

Corticosteroids modify enzyme activity in the synthesis of proteins. These drugs are used to treat Crohn's disease, Addison's disease, COPD, lupus erythematosus, myelomas, and head trauma. The main effect is inhibiting the inflammatory as well as immune responses. Common adverse effects include hypokalemia, hypocalcemia, and hyperglycemia. Corticosteroids also interact with many herbal preparations such as juniper, ginseng, and echinacea.

A is incorrect because corticosteroids do not increase potassium.

D is incorrect because corticosteroids do not directly affect magnesium.

F is incorrect because corticosteroids do not directly affect the hematocrit.

96. A patient has orders for wound care, including antiseptic application. The nurse knows which of the following are accurate regarding antiseptic use? <u>Select all that apply.</u>

    A. Antiseptics can be used on living tissue
    B. Antiseptics sterilize wound surfaces
    C. Antiseptics can be used to kill microorganisms on inanimate objects
    D. Allergies must be assessed before antiseptic use

E. Antiseptics inhibit microorganism growth when placed on wound surfaces

Rationale:

Correct answer: A, D, E

Antiseptics inhibit microorganism growth but do not kill them. Antiseptics have a lower potency than disinfectants. Patient allergies must always be verified before applying antiseptics.

B is incorrect because antiseptics do not sterilize.

C is incorrect because antiseptics can only be applied to living tissue.

97. The healthcare provider suggested a patient take over-the-counter methylcellulose for constipation. The nurse informs the patient of adverse effects, which include what? <u>Select all that apply.</u>

    A. Electrolyte imbalances
    B. Decreased absorption of vitamins
    C. Gas formation
    D. Darkened stools
    E. Discolored urine

Rationale:

Correct answer: A, C

Methylcellulose is a bulk-forming laxative that absorbs excess water from the intestine into the stool to promote peristalsis. With the movement of water into the intestines, electrolytes may follow, leading to a risk for electrolyte imbalances. A naturally occurring substance in methylcellulose is psyllium, which contributes to gas formation and bloating.

B is incorrect because vitamin absorption is not affected by methylcellulose.

D is incorrect because methylcellulose does not affect stool color.

E is incorrect because methylcellulose does not affect urine color.

98. The nurse is caring for a patient with a stage IV pressure ulcer. The nurse knows that the patient would benefit from which of the following supplements for wound healing? Select all that apply.

    A. Vitamin K
    B. Vitamin B1
    C. Zinc
    D. Calcium
    E. Vitamin C

Rationale:

Correct answer: C, E

Vitamin C plays a key role in collagen synthesis, maintenance of connective tissue, and tissue repair, as well as aiding in resistance to infections. Zinc is important for tissue growth, repair, and wound healing.

A is incorrect because Vitamin K plays a role in blood clotting, not wound healing.

B is incorrect because Vitamin B1 plays a role in energy production, not wound healing.

D is incorrect because calcium is important for bone growth and repair and electrolyte balance, not wound healing.

99. The nurse is preparing to administer iron sucrose to a patient. Which of the following interventions are correct for this medication? Select all that apply.

   A. Administer a smaller test dose
   B. Give by deep IM injection using Z-track method
   C. Large doses are given intravenously over 2.5 to 3.5 hours
   D. Monitor for hypertension
   E. Monitor for hypotension

Rationale:

Correct answer: C, E

Iron sucrose is an injectable product for iron-deficiency anemia treatment in those with iron-deficiency and renal disease. Iron sucrose is infused in large doses over 2.5 to 3.5 hours. Patients should be monitored for hypotension when administering iron sucrose.

A is incorrect because a test dose is not required.

B is incorrect because iron sucrose is not given by deep IM injection. The z-track method is used for administering dark-colored solutions that can stain the skin, such as iron-dextran, haloperidol, and Vistaril.

D is incorrect because hypertension is not an adverse effect of iron sucrose.

100. The nurse is preparing an administration of omeprazole to a patient. Which of the following actions should be followed for administration of a proton pump inhibitor (PPI)? Select all that apply.

    A. PPI should be taken on an empty stomach
    B. PPI should be taken with meals
    C. PPI should not be crushed or chewed
    D. Open the capsule and chew contents for best absorption

E. PPI should be taken only when heartburn occurs

Rationale:

Correct answer: A, C

PPI are anti-secretory agents that will bind to proton pumps or hydrogen ion pumps in the GI tract. The outcome is decreased production of gastric acid secretion. These are given for erosive esophagitis, symptomatic GERD, ulcers, and stress ulcer prophylaxis. For best effects, the PPI should be given on an empty stomach, and the pills should not be chewed or crushed.

B is incorrect because taking the PPI with meals will affect the absorption of the medication.

D is incorrect because the pills should not be opened, chewed, or crushed.

E is incorrect because PPI should be taken regularly to prevent the production of gastric acid. Bedtime doses suppress nocturnal gastric acid production.